new
pregnancy
and birth

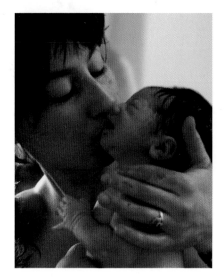

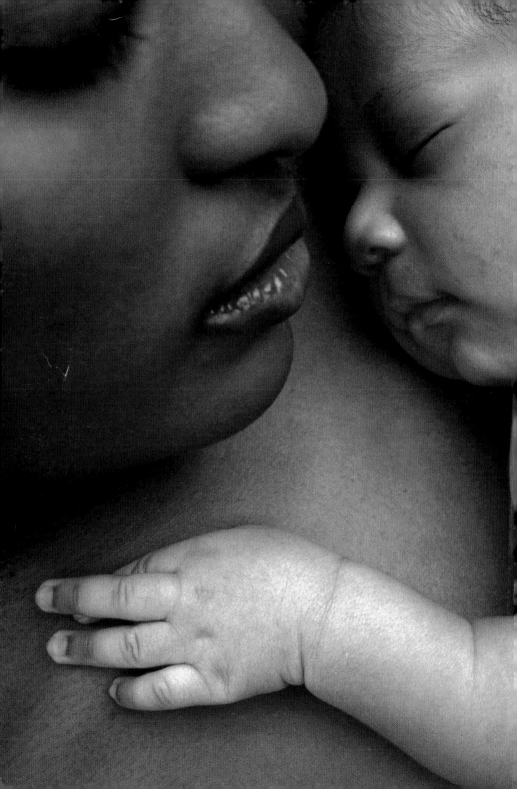

new pregnancy and birth

DRmiriam stoppard

MD FRCP

LONDON, NEW YORK, MUNICH, MELBOURNE, DELHI

For Maggie and Evie, my darling identical twin granddaughters

Produced for Dorling Kindersley by **Cooling Brown**
Design **Arthur Brown, Peter Cooling, Tish Jones, Juliette Norsworthy**
Editorial **Jemima Dunne**

Dorling Kindersley
Consultant Editor **Jinny Johnson**
Managing Editors **Penny Warren, Esther Ripley**
Managing Art Editor **Marianne Markham**
Editor **Emma Maule**
Senior Designers **Nicola Rodway, Anne Fisher**
Production Editor **Ben Marcus**
Production Controller **Alice Holloway**
Creative Technical Support **Sonia Charbonnier**
Jacket Designer **Charlotte Seymour**

First published by Dorling Kindersley in 1985
This revised edition published in Great Britain in 2009 by
Dorling Kindersley Limited, 80 Strand, London WC2 0RL
A Penguin Company

A CIP catalogue record is available from the British Library.
ISBN: 978-1-4053-35188

First reproduced in Singapore by Colourscan;
this revised edition reproduced in London by Altaimage
Printed in China by L-Rex

Discover more at
www.dk.com

Approaching motherhood

For many women today motherhood comes rather later in life than it used to. In the UK, the average age for a first baby is now 29, compared with 25 only a decade ago, and many women leave starting a family until they are well into their thirties. With improvements to overall maternal health, doctors and midwives are used to dealing with first-time mothers in their late thirties and even mid-forties as a matter of routine. This revised edition of my book takes account of this as well as the latest developments in medical research and hospital practices.

Women nowadays work for most of their pregnancy. This means that the planning for a modern pregnancy and the birth is quite different from that in the past. Now most women want to give careful consideration to their future job security and I have outlined the advantages and disadvantages in this book of combining work, pregnancy and motherhood. But no one knows before the birth of their own child just how they will feel after the event. Even if you have arranged to start working again after, say, six months, you may find it impossible to leave your baby and decide to wait for a few months longer.

Every woman is beset by doubts, fears and anxieties – you wouldn't be normal if you weren't. Yet it will all seem easy in retrospect. Meanwhile, it's reassuring to think about the women all around you who are enjoying pregnancies, having memorable labours and births and, despite some sleepless nights, are thrilled with their babies. You, like them, will find that pregnancy and birth introduce you to the most fulfilling phase of your life.

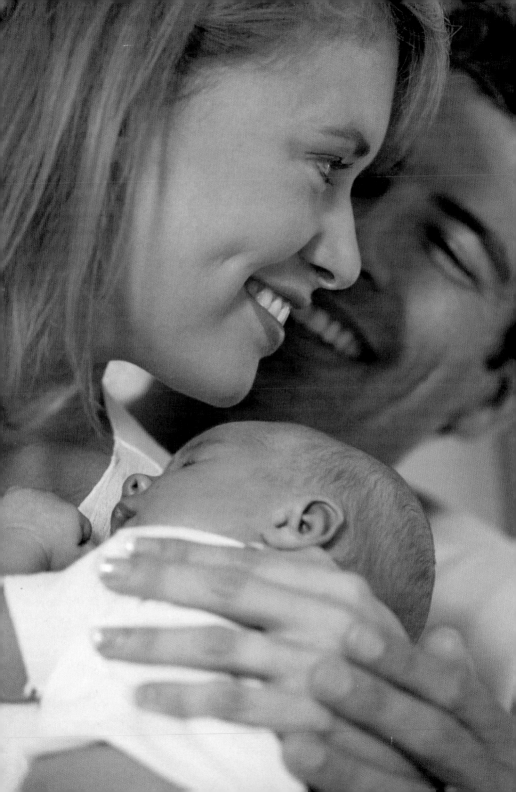

Contents

Introduction

It's been a long time since I wrote my first book on pregnancy and childbirth and much has changed since then. One of the most important and welcome changes is the switch from doctor-supervised pregnancy and labour to one in which midwives play a major role.

Midwife teams

The concept of the "team" midwife is now adopted everywhere. Within this scheme of working, you will be seen by the same group of midwives during your antenatal care, your labour and postnatal recovery, making pregnancy and hospital birth a happier and more relaxed experience than it's been in the past. Women, midwives and doctors all benefit from this scheme as mothers are able to get to know the midwives in the team during their pregnancy and so feel more confident and secure. High standards of care among so many skilled hands is assured and now that there are so many normal births, doctors are free to handle the more complicated ones that need their attention.

Diagnostic tests

Technology has moved fast. Chorionic villus sampling and ultrasound scanning techniques have become so sophisticated that the majority of women who need it can benefit from the early diagnostic information they can supply. This means that a woman whose baby is at risk of inheriting a chromosomal or genetic disorder can be diagnosed within the first ten to 12 weeks of pregnancy and, if she wishes, can opt for an early and safer termination than was possible in the past.

Fetal medicine is also so advanced that in some centres a problem such as a heart defect or blood disorder can be detected and treated in the uterus. However, the morality of these interventions continues to be a matter of fierce debate.

More and more information is now available about maintaining the health of pregnant women and we are aware of the health hazards of food-borne diseases that can affect the fetus. Women are being warned to be meticulous, not only about what they eat, but also how they prepare their food.

Know your options

Pregnancy, labour and birth ought to be joyful experiences for a woman and her partner and above all else I hope this book will help you both to feel really positive about pregnancy and birth. For this to happen, it is important to know what options do exist. Armed with this knowledge you will find the confidence and enthusiasm to ask questions and get the information you need in order to exercise your options and make choices

The first weeks
Learning starts from the moment your baby's born, and the steepest part of a baby's learning curve is during the all-important first six weeks.

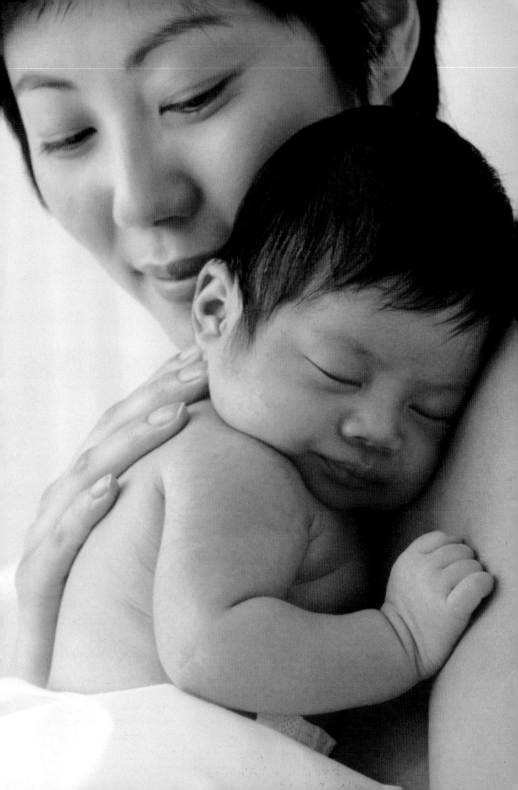

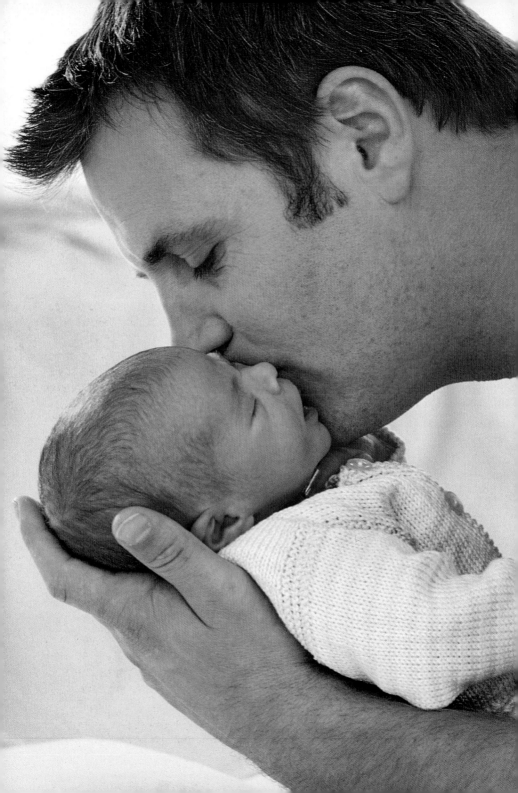

that suit you. This book aims to outline the options that lie before you, and then, having decided on what suits you, to give you the confidence to try to get the delivery and birth you want. I have included not only useful information to help you to have a reasoned discussion with a doctor or midwife, but also given you lists of possible questions to ask when you are choosing a hospital.

My other aim in writing this book is to remove fear and mystery by presenting information about pregnancy and birth as openly and objectively as I can. It's been known for decades that fear of the unknown in pregnancy has a direct effect on labour and delivery; it causes pain, discomfort and slow, difficult labours. If, on the other hand, a woman has been trained during her pregnancy to listen to and observe her body, to read its messages, to act with them, particularly with breathing techniques, relaxation exercises and pelvic muscle exercises, she can help make the birth less painful, a great deal more comfortable and a truly joyful event.

Fathers

There is much research to show that if men are involved from the moment pregnancy is confirmed they become active and enthusiastic fathers. This means being involved in all the preparations, and in antenatal classes and clinics, in decisions as to where and how to have the baby, and with the care of the baby from day one.

Father's role
Get to know your baby by holding her close and talking to her. Carry your baby around in a sling and try to be there for feeds, changing and bathtime.

If men are shut out at any stage, the role of father is more difficult to assimilate. There is no greater help to a pregnant woman than an interested and sympathetic partner. There is no better attendant in the delivery room than an understanding, supportive father – although you might also like to have a close relative or friend – and there's no better help with a newborn baby than an active, passionate dad. The labour itself can be just as remarkable an experience for the father, as the following letter testifies.

One father's experience
"Regardless of where your baby is being born, at home or in hospital, be prepared to leave your sense of embarrassment somewhere else – you'll soon realize that what is happening to your partner is the most real thing she's ever experienced. She may groan and moan softly or loudly, become totally uninterested in you, ask you questions you have no answers for ('How much longer?').

"Since your partner's putting her whole self into the labour, it will help her and you if you become as totally involved as possible. You can help her greatly by answering the questions the midwives ask and by making the decisions – she's in no state to think about anything but what is happening to her body – and above all by being positive. Never cast even a shadow of doubt into her mind. Always tell her that she's doing well, because, no matter what she is doing, she's doing the best she can. Do not judge her – help her, give her some of your energy. The amount of togetherness that you discover during the birth of your child will remain with you and grow for the rest of your lives."

1 Deciding to have a baby

The professor of obstetrics at my medical school used to tell us that there was no right time to have a baby because something else always came up in a couple's professional or domestic life. The corollary of this is that there's no wrong time to have a baby either. Paramount in the decision to have a baby, however, is that it is wanted; ideally it should also be planned. Even planning is often not as perfect as we would like nor, in my opinion, should it be. For one thing, couples may not find it easy to conceive once they have made the decision, so be prepared for the best planning to go awry.

Are you healthy enough?

Every year a small number of babies are born who are not as healthy as they might be. There are many reasons why this may happen, but two of the most important are the nutrition and fitness of the mother. Although it has been noted that maternal malnutrition and lack of fitness become more common as you descend the economic scale, it is also worth bearing in mind that eating disorders or excessive dieting may also affect your health. Try to pay attention to nutrition and lifestyle as well as your general state of health before you decide to have a baby (see p.110).

Diet

If you're not already doing so, you can improve your health enormously by examining your diet. You may think you eat well but take a closer look. Do you skip breakfast and eat a small lunch, saving your appetite for an evening meal? Do you leave the fresh fruit for your children? Do you resort to high-calorie snacks to get you through the day? You can improve your health almost immediately by increasing your intake of fresh fruit, vegetables and high-fibre foods, and cutting out highly refined, starchy foods (see pp.106–114).

Folic acid

One of the B group of vitamins, folic acid (folate is the natural form) helps to reduce the risk of spinal abnormalities in the fetus. Take folic acid supplements for at least three months before you start trying for a baby (400mcg per day is the recommended dose), and at least 12 weeks into your pregnancy. The supplements bought over the counter are fine for most women. Eat plenty of foods rich in folate such as dark-green leafy vegetables, bread, cereals and

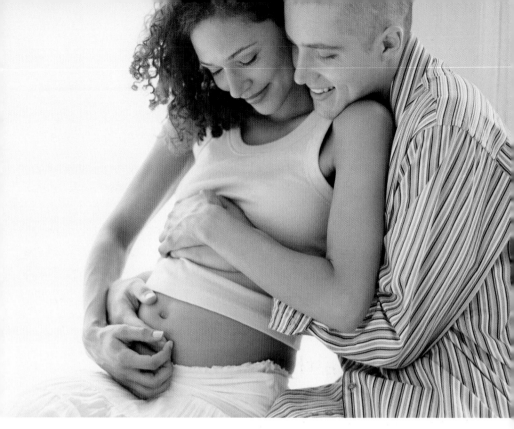

some nuts (but avoid peanuts). If your baby was unplanned, start taking folic acid as soon as you find out you're pregnant.

Exercise

Try to take some exercise, either a sport such as tennis, swimming or jogging, or start an exercise programme using a rowing machine, an exercise bike, or simply take a brisk walk. Try to exercise for 30 minutes at least four times a week, during which you should aim to get slightly out of breath and sweat a little.

Smoking, alcohol and drugs

You should take particular care to give up "social" drugs before you conceive, including cigarettes (*see p.115*). Smoking is associated with infertility in women,

For the health for your baby
It's important for both you and your partner to eat a good balanced diet, take plenty of exercise and find the time to relax together to improve your chances of having a healthy baby.

although its effect on male fertility may be more damaging. Sperm are more at risk than eggs from the chemicals in cigarette smoke, and it is believed that smoking could cause damage to chromosomes in the cells of smokers.

The risks of smoking to the unborn baby are well documented. It is now known that passive smoking can be as harmful as smoking itself; a woman living with people who smoke inhales a lot of nicotine and tars from the cigarette smoke in the air around her.

New research suggests that alcohol is riskier at the time of conception and during the early weeks than was previously thought. Alcohol is increasingly being linked to certain birth defects and, in severe cases, to a syndrome producing physical and mental abnormalities (see p.116). To be on the safe side, avoid drinking alcohol altogether if you are trying for a baby.

It is also risky to take recreational drugs in pregnancy. Cannabis is known to interfere with the normal production of male sperm and increases the risk of conceiving a baby with chromosomal abnormalities. It is also thought that LSD can cause birth defects if taken around the time of conception.

Age of the parents

This will always be a factor for you to consider when deciding to have a baby but may not be as decisive as you might think. Considerations of personal freedom and career moves are causing more and more women to wait until they are over 30 to become pregnant, but many still fear that they may be leaving it too late. This is because they may have heard that the longer they wait the greater is the chance of having a difficult pregnancy or even, possibly, a child with an abnormality. However, although the risk of having a baby with Down's syndrome, for example, increases with the age of the mother (see p.79), carefully documented case studies show that it is not physically dangerous to the woman herself if she defers pregnancy until she is past her twenties.

The risks undoubtedly increase with age but every decision to have a child is unique and the age of the parents is only one factor, and a very small one, in weighing up the risks and benefits. The age of the father relates more to infertility than to a risk factor. Many other factors affect the risk factor ratio in each woman's case. Of course, what these statistics do is to band all mothers over the age of 30 together, regardless of their health or financial background, whereas an important factor in maternal risk is the mother's socio-economic situation. The complications during pregnancy and delivery for this group are not related to age but to other factors such as malnutrition;

RUBELLA

If your developing baby is exposed to the rubella virus (German measles), malformations, including deafness, blindness and heart disease, may occur. This is particularly likely during the first three months, when all the vital organs are forming and developing.

What to do

If you did not have rubella as a child and were not vaccinated against it at puberty, consult your doctor before you try for a baby and ask for a blood test to find out if you're immune. If you aren't immune, ask to be vaccinated against the disease, and then wait at least three months before trying to conceive. If you're already pregnant, a blood test will show if you have some immunity.

However, even if vaccinated you may not be completely immune so if you come into contact with the disease, tell your doctor at once, though unfortunately contact is most hazardous before the rash appears. If you are infected, you may want to discuss the difficult decision about whether to terminate your pregnancy.

an individual pregnant woman will only need special care if she is poorly nourished, regardless of her age *(see p.12)*.

Bear in mind, too, that although physically a woman may be better suited to childbirth in her early twenties, she may not be ready to be a parent emotionally or financially. When she is younger a woman may be too involved with her career to have children, or she may not have met the right person to be the father of her children.

Although fertility does diminish with age *(see p.22)*, an important factor to consider is that, statistically speaking, the odds are greatly in favour of you having a successful pregnancy at almost any age provided you are healthy. Many studies have been done on normal pregnancies in women past the age of 40 and all of them have concluded that the general health of the mother is much more important than age alone as a factor in predicting how the pregnancy will turn out – so remember if your health is good, the decision to have a baby should not be abandoned on account of age alone.

Pre-existing medical conditions

Some pre-existing medical conditions – including diabetes, heart disease and Rhesus incompatibility *(see pp.154–161)* – may cause problems in pregnancy. Even so, with careful antenatal care you may still be able to give birth normally. If you have a long-standing medical condition or if you are taking any medication regularly, you need to discuss the possibility of a pregnancy with your doctor. If you're having long-term drug treatment – for example, for epilepsy – talk to your doctor before trying for a baby.

HIV/AIDS

It is important that you know how to protect yourself against the HIV virus that leads to AIDS, and to be assertive about it. All women should insist on safe sex and any new sexual encounter should be prefaced by a frank discussion about HIV/AIDS. Over three-quarters of women who become infected with the HIV virus acquire it through sexual intercourse, there being no particular social pattern. The risk varies from person to person and partner to partner – some women do not become infected after hundreds of contacts, while others are infected after one.

When a virus gets into the body the blood makes a substance called an antibody. People who have been infected with HIV produce antibodies to the virus and, when tested, are said to be HIV positive. Because the mother's antibodies can cross the placenta, all babies born to HIV positive mothers will also show up as HIV positive initially, but not all of these babies will be infected with the virus. Some time between the ages of six and 18 months many babies will lose their mothers' antibodies and, once tested as HIV negative, they are then presumed to be uninfected.

More sensitive tests are now being used to allow a diagnosis of HIV infection to be made in the first few months of life. Even if the baby is found to be HIV positive, a good many babies survive into later childhood, although a third of HIV positive babies die before the age of two.

HIV testing is now offered (and recommended) to all pregnant women. If you are found to be HIV positive, you should be counselled about the likelihood of contracting full-blown AIDS, and also about your own risk of transmitting the virus to the baby. There are now treatments available that reduce the risk of a mother infecting her baby.

Effects on lifestyle

A survey done in the US showed that the number of women who considered motherhood the most pleasurable aspect of being a woman had dropped in the last 20 years, while the number of women who opted for work as being more fulfilling had risen. As women in the West have re-examined their status in society and decided to be more self-determined than they have been in the past, aided by reliable contraceptive methods, fewer are taking the role of wife and mother as the automatic choice in life. The investment of more time in the pursuit of a career also means that more women are opting to have families later in their lives.

For most women, having children is now a matter of choice and planning, and their decision to be a mother is a well considered one, although unfortunately too many teenage girls still become pregnant by accident. Nowadays, few people would subscribe to the unquestioned idealization of the act of childbearing that once made society view it as essential to women's fulfilment.

Some women, as they get older and fear that their fertility is diminishing, regard single parenthood as a possible choice, even though they may not have found a partner with whom they wish to settle down. Women who make this decision and conceive a baby are usually remarkable for their single-mindedness and are quite prepared to face the implications of being a lone mother. To them motherhood is a chosen state, not one imposed by chance.

Anxiety about parenthood

When you consider the change in lifestyle, the possible disruption of a happy relationship, the concessions and adjustments that have to be made with the arrival of a baby, the decision to remain childless becomes more understandable than it might have been. Many people fear

STOPPING CONTRACEPTION

If you are taking the oral contraceptive pill, you may decide to have two or three normal menstrual periods before you become pregnant. During the intervening months you could use some mechanical form of contraception such as condoms, or a cap or diaphram (*see p.235*).

Much has been written about a woman's return to fertility after she has been taking the pill, particularly for long periods of time. Originally it was thought that fertility was increased after stopping the pill as the body overcompensated for long periods of suppressed fertility. We now know that this is not necessarily so, but most women conceive in the first year after stopping the pill and nearly all women after two years. If you suspect that you have become pregnant while taking the pill, check with your doctor at once as there can be a slight risk to the embryo from the hormones in the oral contraceptive pill.

There's no need to put off conception after having an IUCD (coil) removed. If you become pregnant with one in place, your doctor won't try to remove it as it may be difficult, and the risk of precipitating a miscarriage is greater than if it is left in place.

parenthood and it's a reasonable anxiety. It's natural to worry about coping with your child's upbringing.

There may be economic pressures, the problem of resuming your career and possible frustration due to loss of freedom. Not everyone relishes the fact that they are no longer free agents and you'd be quite normal if you questioned your ability to feel loving and caring towards your baby all the time. In normal life you are besieged by many negative feelings such as resentment, bad temper, or frustration, and there's no reason to think that the presence of your baby will call an end to these feelings.

It is perhaps only when you become a parent that you realize how much is demanded of you. In the early years all the giving must come from you. But the one lesson that I have learned is that the more you give, the more is given back to you as your child grows older.

A father's role

The role of the modern father has changed too. The majority of fathers take the responsibility of being a parent very seriously and they are not prepared to be strangers to their children. For many years men were shut out of pregnancy and from the day-to-day care of their children on the assumption that it was woman's work and not their place to interfere. But now liberated mothers have fostered liberated fathers. These fathers feel free to indulge all their paternal instincts, and they want to be involved with their partners during pregnancy and delivery and are not prepared to miss out on their children growing up. The modern father is an active father rather than a passive one.

Even in the early years your child will reward you with irreplaceable moments of pleasure, possibly pride, and as she grows older, with more and more hours of companionship, love, comfort and joy. Most fathers who take a keen interest in the pregnancy stay interested after the baby is born.

Studies have shown that a father becomes more closely attached to his baby according to how much he holds her during the first six weeks of life and whether or not he answers the baby's cry. His attitude is also affected by his partner's enjoyment of pregnancy and motherhood. The happier a man is about his partner's pregnancy, the more he shares in the monitoring of her antenatal care, and the more he looks forward to enjoying fatherhood, the more he will get out of the first few weeks of his baby's life.

Sharing responsibilities

Most couples agree that parents should be equal and the roles of parenting and childrearing must be shared, if possible. When you make the decision to have a baby you and your partner should view it as a contract: a contract holding you both equally responsible for rearing the child you have conceived.

Try to discuss and agree with each other about the roles you're going to play. No longer are women willing to be the sole carer, confined to the house while the father leaves home early to work and doesn't return until the baby is fast asleep. These are some of the issues that must be resolved between you before your baby is born if you want to provide a happy and stable environment for your child.

Becoming pregnant

Knowing about your natural body cycles will give you enough information both to conceive and to avoid conception. The body rhythms that you can observe are your monthly menstrual cycles and the appearance and consistency of the cervical mucus (your vaginal discharge).

Observing body rhythms

Although many women have regular 28-day cycles, some have menstrual cycles of varying length. After recording your menstrual cycles, say for four months, you may find that the shortest one was 26 days and the longest one was 32 days. In this case, the fertile days could be from the 9th to the 21st day of each cycle, since ovulation normally occurs 14 days before menstruation, and the sperm can live for three or four days within the woman's body. For conception, these are the days to concentrate on.

Your vaginal discharge (mucus) goes through a cycle of changes as the month progresses. Just after menstruation there is hardly any mucus, but it is cloudy, sticky and thick. As you approach the fertile period it becomes abundant, clear and stretchy. As soon as you notice this change you've entered your fertile period. Fertility wanes when the mucus becomes cloudy, sticky and thick once again.

INFLUENCE OF CHROMOSOMES AND GENES

Each cell in the body contains 46 chromosomes in 23 pairs, one half of each pair comes from the sperm and the other half from the ovum. Each chromosome consists of two chains (known as the double helix) of thousands of genes strung together.

Gender

One pair of the 23 pairs of chromosomes determines gender. This pair is either XX (female) or XY (male), made up from donations from the mother and father. A mother only donates an X chromosome in her eggs, but a father can donate either X or Y, because a man produces two kinds of sperm – X (female) or Y (male). Biologically the male is responsible for the sex of the baby. If a Y sperm unites with the ovum, the baby will be a boy (XY) but if it's an X, the baby will be a girl (XX). Scientists have discovered that the Y sperm is produced in greater numbers, has a longer tail and moves faster than the X sperm, but the X sperm survives longer. Although there's no proof, some say that if you want a boy, you should have sex as near as possible to the day you ovulate; and for a girl, a few days before.

Genes direct development

A gene is a minute unit of DNA (deoxyribo-nucleic acid). Genes direct the development of all the body's organs and systems and determine our intellectual and physical characteristics. Characteristics such as the colour of the eyes and hair have a gene from the mother and father. Each characteristic has a dominant and recessive form. The gene for dark hair, for example, is always dominant over the gene for blond hair, and the gene for brown eyes will always dominate the one for blue. However, both genes are present, though one is masked, so two dark-haired parents can have a blond child whose hair colour is represented by the masked blond from each parent.

Frequency of intercourse

Your chances of conceiving a baby are not helped by frequent intercourse. The more often a man ejaculates the less sperm is contained in his ejaculate. However, the quality (motility) of the sperm may be more important than the actual numbers.

If you're trying for a baby, it's a good idea for your partner to abstain from ejaculation for a few days before your fertile period to allow sperm numbers to rise, then to have intercourse no more than once daily during your fertile days.

If you tend to have an extremely irregular menstrual cycle, however, it may be difficult to be sure exactly when your fertile days are in order to have intercourse at the right time. Check with your doctor and ask for advice on this.

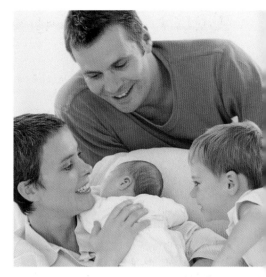

Genetic inheritance
Children inherit a variety of physical characteristics from each of their parents.

Genetic counselling

Quite rightly, emphasis is put on the mother's health because it is crucial to give the baby a healthy environment in which to develop. But the health of the father is important too. If either the sperm or the egg is defective, they may not be able to unite at all, leading to some causes of infertility. If sperm are only slightly defective it is possible for a baby to develop that is not completely normal.

Some conditions are due to abnormalities of the chromosomes. Chromosome counts may give you some idea of the likelihood of conceiving a child who will suffer from the disease. This simple, painless procedure involves some cells being gently scraped from the inside of your mouth. The cells are then examined under a microscope.

Every year thousands of children are born with congenital malformations, but the majority of these cannot be anticipated. Genetic defects are not related to general health. Some conditions due to

chromosome abnormalities such as Down's syndrome occur at fertilization so parents cannot be tested beforehand. If there's a history of a disease or condition in either partner that runs through family members and generations, then you should seek genetic counselling and testing. Conditions that run in families include haemophilia, cystic fibrosis, sickle-cell disease and muscular dystrophy and tests are available for these.

Everyone takes some risk, albeit a minute one, when they decide to have a baby, and pregnancy is by no means ruled out if you or your partner have an hereditary tendency to a particular condition. Your decision to go ahead and try can only be helped by having a specialist investigation and counselling to determine the risk, depending on whether the affected gene is recessive (as with cystic fibrosis, for example) or dominant (Huntington's chorea). Speak to your doctor to find out about your options.

Fertilization

If your menstrual cycle is regular, as a general rule fertilization happens about one week after you have finished menstruating or 14 days before your next period begins. About seven to 10 days after this, the fertilized ovum is implanted in the lining of the womb. By the end of another week it is firmly attached by its primitive placenta, which links the developing embryo to its mother (*see p.81*). The placenta is the organ through which foodstuffs and oxygen are carried from the mother to the baby and waste substances are carried from the baby to the mother. It is absolutely crucial to the

healthy progress of pregnancy because it produces the pregnancy hormones that are responsible for maintaining the health of the developing baby, the uterus and the female genital organs. These same hormones also prepare the woman's body for labour and for birth.

The ovum is usually fertilized about a third of the way along the Fallopian tube by a single sperm that was deposited, along with millions of others, in the vagina after ejaculation. Within a few seconds of ejaculation the sperm become mobile with the lashings of their whiplike tails.

The ovum (egg) travels one-third of the way along the Fallopian tube, where it is fertilized

The fertilized egg (now called a zygote) keeps on dividing as it travels down the Fallopian tube

The ovum (egg) is released from its follicle

Seven days after fertilization, the egg (now a ball of cells), implants itself in the uterus lining, and starts to develop into an embryo

Ovarian cycle
Each month the ovary is stimulated by a hormone – follicle-stimulating hormone (FSH) – to ripen an egg. The egg is released around the 14th day of the menstrual cycle and may be fertilized. If it is not fertilized, it passes out of the body through the vagina with the womb lining at your next menstrual period.

This then carries them at top speed out of the acid conditions of the vagina and through the neck of the cervix, which has become more fluid during ovulation, into the cavity of the uterus. In a few seconds the sperm pass through the uterus and enter the Fallopian tube to meet the ovum that is travelling down the tube towards them. Sperm are chemically attracted to the comparatively enormous ovum and attach themselves to it like limpets over the whole surface. However, only one sperm pierces the outer coat of the ovum. Instantly the egg loses its attraction, hardens its outer shell and all the superfluous sperm let go. This whole process, from ejaculation to fertilization, can take less than 60 minutes.

A ripe ovum survives for a maximum of 24 hours; the sooner it is fertilized after release from the follicle, the better. Sperm retain the power to fertilize for three or four days. Fertilization is therefore most likely to occur in the 7–10 days following the end of a period.

Beginning of life

Only the head of the sperm fuses with the ovum, forming a single cell. The cell divides into two in the first 24 hours; by the fourth day it is a ball of over 100 cells. This ball of cells floats free for the first three days in the cavity of the uterus, nurtured on "milk" secreted by glands in the uterine wall. By the end of the first week, it has implanted into the uterine lining, where it is continuously bathed in a lake of its mother's blood, allowing food and waste to pass to and fro. Until week eight the baby is known as an embryo, after which it's called a fetus, Latin for "young one".

CONCEPTION OF TWINS

When a single egg released from the ovary is fertilized and divides into two cells which then separate, this results in the development of identical twins; they are always the same sex and usually share the same placenta. More common are fraternal twins (70 per cent of twins). These occur when two separate eggs are fertilized by two different sperm. Fraternal twins usually have separate placentas and amniotic sacs.

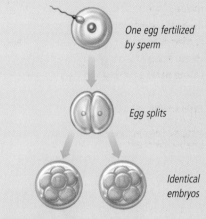

One egg fertilized by sperm

Egg splits

Identical embryos

Identical twins
Once the egg has been fertilized it splits into separate cells. This split may occur after implantation in the uterus.

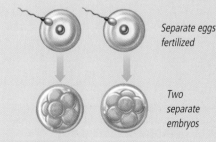

Separate eggs fertilized

Two separate embryos

Fraternal twins
Most twins occur when two eggs are released into the Fallopian tube and each one is fertilized by a separate sperm.

Infertility

Out of about ten million women of childbearing age in Great Britain, around one million are subfertile and unable to have babies. This ratio of one in ten is fairly constant throughout the Western nations. Infertility, however, is not a matter of either partner exclusively but of the couple as a unit. In some circumstances the high fertility of one partner can compensate for the low fertility of the other.

On the other hand, marginal fertility in both partners may result in their failing to get pregnant. This explains the paradox of a childless couple splitting up and then both partners producing children once in a new partnership.

Female infertility

In women one of the most important factors that affects fertility is age. Fertility begins to diminish after the age of 25, but this only becomes significant over the age of 37 or so. The decline in a man's fertility is more gradual. It is the same as a woman's at the age of 20 and wanes slowly to ten per cent by the age of 60.

The barriers to fertility can be physical, psychological or emotional. Many people find the subject difficult to discuss but if as a couple you wish to have your subfertility investigated, you're going to need help, which means you both discussing sensitive subjects in an open and sensible way.

Examining a woman's fertility may involve some or all of the following procedures. Some are time-consuming and invasive, so they are usually deferred until you have been trying to conceive for over a year. Initially, your partner's sperm count and quality are checked.

- Discussion of frequency and type of sexual intercourse.
- Blood tests at the beginning and in the second half of your cycle.
- Surgical exploration, usually laparoscopy, in which a telescope-like instrument is passed through the abdominal wall to allow the doctor to look at your reproductive organs.
- Alternatively, hysterosalpingography (HSG) – X-ray examination of the Fallopian tubes. A fine tube is placed inside the cervix and dye that can be seen on X-ray is injected so any damage or blockage can be seen.

Drug treatment

Women who have very irregular or absent periods may need help to ovulate regularly. All drug treatments aim to stimulate the ovary to produce eggs and run the risk of several eggs being released simultaneously, with an increased risk of multiple pregnancy. The risk is lowest with oral drugs such as clomiphene or tamoxifen. These tend to be used first for a maximum of six months and the woman is monitored by scans or timed blood tests.

If this fails, injection therapy with synthetic hormones (human menopausal gonadotrophin/hMG and human chorionic gonadotrophin/hCG) can be an option. This treatment is monitored by ultrasound and/or blood tests. It can cause the ovaries to swell in which case the treatment has to be abandoned.

Male infertility

In men there are two main causes of infertility: a blockage in the tubes between the testes and the penis, and inadequate production of sperm. Both of these problems require hospital investigation and laboratory tests before they can be excluded. Inadequate sperm production can be one or all of three kinds of deficiency: a low sperm count, low sperm mobility or large numbers of abnormal sperm. These characteristics have to be reported by the laboratory and interpreted by your doctor.

Assisted conception

The ability to assist infertile couples to conceive and give birth to healthy babies has greatly improved with the availability of artificial insemination and in vitro fertilization (IVF).

In artificial insemination, a partner's sperm (artificial insemination by partner, or AIP) or a donor's sperm (donor insemination, or DI) is introduced into the cervix from a syringe. Insemination is done just before or during ovulation. DI may be considered when a man has a very low sperm count, is sterile or is known to be a carrier of or have an hereditary abnormality. DI is also an option for single women who want to have a baby.

Anyone contemplating IVF should know that it's physically and emotionally very demanding and stressful. You need counselling before and during treatment and this is available at all IVF clinics.

For IVF to work, two things are necessary. First, eggs from the female partner, collected after clomiphene or hMG/hCG treatment, and second, sperm from the male partner. Both can be obtained from donors. The eggs are fertilized outside the womb and kept in an incubator for 48 hours, by which time each will have divided into about four cells. One or two embryos can then be transferred into the woman's uterus. Further embryos can be stored.

Occasionally the egg and sperm are placed together in the Fallopian tube, but as this requires a general anaesthetic and a laparoscopy it is less common. Success rates for IVF do depend on the age of the mother and the reason for the treatment in the first place.

HAZARDS AT WORK

If you or your partner work with certain chemicals, lead or radiation, your fertility could be affected. It is now known that certain industrial substances can damage sperm and cause malformed babies and spontaneous miscarriage. If you're not sure about the chemicals or other substances that you work with and how they might affect your chances of conception, ask your doctor, union representative or human resources manager. Only a relatively small number of substances have been recognized as needing a safety threshold. However, this safe level of exposure doesn't take into account how the chemicals may affect fertility. Rather than taking a chance, if one of you works with a hazardous substance, you might consider trying to change your job before conceiving a baby. If that's not possible and you can't avoid contact with doubtful substances, follow stringent safety regulations, wear protective clothing, and avoid breathing in dust or fumes and skin contact with the substance.

2 Finding out you are pregnant

There are two quite separate aspects to finding out you're pregnant. The first is about confirming your pregnancy; this can be picked up in signs from your body such as nausea, having to empty your bladder more often and dilated veins on the surface of your breasts. The other involves intellectual and emotional acceptance of your pregnancy. The first may be tinged with excitement; the second coloured by feelings of ambivalence. No matter how much you've wanted to be pregnant, you may well have a mixed response to the news that you really are pregnant.

Early symptoms of pregnancy

Perhaps the earliest symptom of pregnancy for many women is the feeling that they really are pregnant. Many women describe a definite consciousness of pregnancy that I believe has as much to do with the first secretion of pregnancy hormones as anything else. These hormones affect your body in every respect, as well as your mind and the way you feel.

Another early sign of pregnancy is fatigue. Although some women feel energized, the majority would confess to feeling tired. However, it is a new kind of tiredness never felt before. Some women say that they find themselves dropping off to sleep at any time of the day; others say that they become so sleepy in the early afternoon that they have to stop what they are doing and wait for the tiredness to pass. Others are tired in the early evening. Whenever it happens, this fatigue is often uncontrollable and you just have to sleep. This condition is known as narcolepsy.

I've never found a satisfactory explanation for this overwhelming desire to sleep. It could well be an effect of the hormone progesterone, which reaches high levels in the blood during early pregnancy. Progesterone is a sedative in human beings with powerful tranquillizing and hypnotic effects. It also accounts for the beatific look that is classically associated with pregnancy. There is another type of fatigue that occurs later on in pregnancy (*see p.152*), which is due simply to the physical tiredness of carrying the extra weight.

Missed period
Within two weeks of fertilization you'll miss a period – the classic sign of pregnancy. This is called amenorrhoea.

While pregnancy is the most common cause of amenorrhoea, it's not the only one so don't automatically assume you're pregnant. A severe physical illness, shock, jet lag, surgery, even anxiety, are known to delay a period.

Equally, it's quite common to have a light bleed after the pregnancy is already established, at the time you might normally have had a period. This is why some pregnancies appear only to be eight months in length.

Morning sickness

Nausea, occasionally accompanied by vomiting, occurs from about week six of pregnancy and is often experienced as "morning sickness", although it may happen at other times of the day. It rarely continues beyond the first three months, gradually stopping in that time (see p.148).

Morning sickness is caused by the increasing levels of hormones circulating in the blood, which can directly irritate the lining of the stomach. One hormone, human chorionic gonadotrophin (hCG), is produced to keep up supplies of oestrogen and progesterone to maintain the pregnancy. Its presence in urine confirms a pregnancy (see p.26). The build-up of hCG roughly parallels the time of nausea, tailing off at 12–14 weeks. Hormones also cause a rapid clearing of sugar from the blood, which may result in the simultaneous feeling of hunger and sickness that some women describe.

Tastes and cravings

A change in taste and in preferences for certain foods may be one of the first signs of pregnancy, happening even before you miss a period. It's quite common to go off certain food and drink, especially fried foods, coffee and alcohol. Some women experience a metallic taste in the mouth that affects their appreciation of food. Cravings are thought to be due to the rising hormone levels and are sometimes felt during the second half of the menstrual cycle for the same reason. Try not to indulge cravings for high-calorie foods that are low in nutrients.

Frequency of urination

As the uterus begins to swell, it presses on the bladder. Hormonal changes lead to differences in muscle tone, which also affects the bladder. As a result, it tries to expel even small amounts of urine, and many women notice the need to pass urine more frequently a week after conception.

Unless there's a burning sensation or pain when you pass urine there is no need to consult your doctor about frequency of urination (micturition). Around week 12, the enlarging uterus rises up out of the pelvic cavity, which reduces the pressure on the bladder for the next few months of your pregnancy.

Breasts

The breast changes in early pregnancy (see p.92) are the result of stimulation by progesterone and these are the first signs some women notice. Even before you miss your first period your nipples will feel sore and your breasts will enlarge and become tender. Veins are prominent over the surface of the breast and the creamy nodules in the nipple area (the areola) will begin to grow. The nipples also start to enlarge and deepen in colour.

Receiving the news

Most of us feel some ambivalence about pregnancy and parenthood and find that our feelings shift with our moods. It's absolutely normal to have mixed feelings. It would be unrealistic to imagine that your life will remain unchanged after the baby comes and it's better to think ahead. Don't feel that you're inadequate for having conflicting feelings and don't try to suppress them. It's far more sensible to acknowledge and face up to them, rather than trying to reach a point where there are no conflicts. Going through pregnancy is a phase of your emotional growth, and at the end of it you should have a better understanding and awareness of yourself.

PREGNANCY TESTS

Detecting the presence of the pregnancy hormone human chorionic gonadotrophin (*see p.25*) in urine is the most common test. This hormone is produced in increasing amounts in the early part of pregnancy.

Home kits
You'll probably prefer to find out whether or not you're pregnant in the privacy of your own home so you're sure of complete confidentiality. Home pregnancy testing kits are at least 99 per cent reliable. It's essential to follow the instructions on the packet exactly, since methods vary from kit to kit. Positive results are rarely wrong, but false negatives may occur if the test is used too early.

Taking the test
Pass a sample of your first urine of the morning into a clean, soap-free container. Don't drink anything before the test as this will dilute the sample. A negative result from a test does not always mean you're not pregnant. If the other signs persist, try again in seven days; you may have tested too early in your pregnancy.

Unexpected results
It is possible that a test will show a positive result that becomes negative when repeated, and your period may start a few days later. Don't worry. Half of all conceptions do not become established pregnancies, as the fertilized egg fails to grow properly in the lining of the uterus and there is a natural termination. The test may have been positive because it was done before the loss of the fertilized egg. To avoid this error, do the test around the time of your first missed period. If there is a weak but positive result, repeat the test a few days later.

Do you have the right result?
A number of factors can affect the accuracy of your pregnancy test results:
- Incorrectly collected or stored urine samples can lead to errors.
- If the test is performed too early, the concentration of human chorionic gonadotrophin (hCG) will be too low to detect. It is important to know when your period was due. Irregular or infrequent periods can affect an accurate indication of pregnancy.
- Fertility drugs containing hCG can change the results. Contraceptive pills, antibiotics and painkillers shouldn't affect results.
- If the equipment used for the test is too hot, the result may be false. Urine must be room temperature at the time of the test.

Different reactions

The reactions to the confirmation of your pregnancy may not be what you expected. It's possible that personal circumstances change so that a pregnancy is unwelcome. A woman may resent a pregnancy taking over her body and feel bitter because her active life is curtailed.

Some women become depressed when they realize they are pregnant and even consider termination. This is painting a negative picture, more negative perhaps than how the majority of women feel. However, the most crucial part of receiving the news that you're pregnant is for you and your partner to accept the pregnancy fully. Don't think that you can ignore it and carry on as normal just because the bump doesn't show for the first few weeks or months. It is important that you both start thinking of your pregnancy realistically, not just in a rosy glow.

HOW TO CALCULATE YOUR ESTIMATED DATE OF DELIVERY (EDD)

The average pregnancy is 266 days long measured from conception, or 280 days measured from the first day of your last menstrual period (LMP). Remember 280 days is average and you may not be average. The possibility of your baby arriving on your EDD depends on your having regular 28-day cycles. All that doctors are prepared to say is that a normal pregnancy may be anywhere between 38 and 42 weeks. To find your EDD, find the date of your LMP in the first row of each section; the date below it is your EDD. Or work it out as follows:

LMP	17.09.09
+ 9 months	17.06.10
+ 7 days	24.06.10

FINDING YOUR ESTIMATED DATE OF DELIVERY

Jan	1	2	3	4	5	6	7	8	9	10	11	12	13	14	15	16	17	18	19	20	21	22	23	24	25	26	27	28	29	30	31
Oct/Nov	8	9	10	11	12	13	14	15	16	17	18	19	20	21	22	23	24	25	26	27	28	29	30	31	1	2	3	4	5	6	7
Feb	1	2	3	4	5	6	7	8	9	10	11	12	13	14	15	16	17	18	19	20	21	22	23	24	25	26	27	28	29	30	31
Nov/Dec	8	9	10	11	12	13	14	15	16	17	18	19	20	21	22	23	24	25	26	27	28	29	30	31	1	2	3	4	5	6	7
Mar	1	2	3	4	5	6	7	8	9	10	11	12	13	14	15	16	17	18	19	20	21	22	23	24	25	26	27	28	29	30	31
Dec/Jan	6	7	8	9	10	11	12	13	14	15	16	17	18	19	20	21	22	23	24	25	26	27	28	29	30	31	1	2	3	4	5
Apr	1	2	3	4	5	6	7	8	9	10	11	12	13	14	15	16	17	18	19	20	21	22	23	24	25	26	27	28	29	30	31
Jan/Feb	6	7	8	9	10	11	12	13	14	15	16	17	18	19	20	21	22	23	24	25	26	27	28	29	30	31	1	2	3	4	5
May	1	2	3	4	5	6	7	8	9	10	11	12	13	14	15	16	17	18	19	20	21	22	23	24	25	26	27	28	29	30	31
Feb/Mar	5	6	7	8	9	10	11	12	13	14	15	16	17	18	19	20	21	22	23	24	25	26	27	28	29	30	31	1	2	3	4
June	1	2	3	4	5	6	7	8	9	10	11	12	13	14	15	16	17	18	19	20	21	22	23	24	25	26	27	28	29	30	31
Mar/Apr	8	9	10	11	12	13	14	15	16	17	18	19	20	21	22	23	24	25	26	27	28	29	30	31	1	2	3	4	5	6	7
July	1	2	3	4	5	6	7	8	9	10	11	12	13	14	15	16	17	18	19	20	21	22	23	24	25	26	27	28	29	30	31
Apr/May	7	8	9	10	11	12	13	14	15	16	17	18	19	20	21	22	23	24	25	26	27	28	29	30	31	1	2	3	4	5	6
Aug	1	2	3	4	5	6	7	8	9	10	11	12	13	14	15	16	17	18	19	20	21	22	23	24	25	26	27	28	29	30	31
May/June	8	9	10	11	12	13	14	15	16	17	18	19	20	21	22	23	24	25	26	27	28	29	30	31	1	2	3	4	5	6	7
Sept	1	2	3	4	5	6	7	8	9	10	11	12	13	14	15	16	17	18	19	20	21	22	23	24	25	26	27	28	29	30	31
June/July	8	9	10	11	12	13	14	15	16	17	18	19	20	21	22	23	24	25	26	27	28	29	30	31	1	2	3	4	5	6	7
Oct	1	2	3	4	5	6	7	8	9	10	11	12	13	14	15	16	17	18	19	20	21	22	23	24	25	26	27	28	29	30	31
July/Aug	8	9	10	11	12	13	14	15	16	17	18	19	20	21	22	23	24	25	26	27	28	29	30	31	1	2	3	4	5	6	7
Nov	1	2	3	4	5	6	7	8	9	10	11	12	13	14	15	16	17	18	19	20	21	22	23	24	25	26	27	28	29	30	31
Aug/Sept	8	9	10	11	12	13	14	15	16	17	18	19	20	21	22	23	24	25	26	27	28	29	30	31	1	2	3	4	5	6	7
Dec	1	2	3	4	5	6	7	8	9	10	11	12	13	14	15	16	17	18	19	20	21	22	23	24	25	26	27	28	29	30	31
Sept/Oct	7	8	9	10	11	12	13	14	15	16	17	18	19	20	21	22	23	24	25	26	27	28	29	30	31	1	2	3	4	5	6

The working woman

In most countries there are laws governing the length of time a woman has to work in order to receive financial benefits (*see pp.247–9*), and the conditions that her employer must meet on her return to work. Outside these laws the majority of employers are keen to cooperate with your plans for discontinuing employment before the birth and for resuming it afterwards. There is usually a statutory period of notice for maternity leave that you must give your employer; if you don't comply with this you may lose benefits, so find out about your rights as early as possible. Towards the end of the first trimester you should be thinking about your future work. If you wish to have your job held open for you after your maternity leave, talk to your employer to see how your plans can be accommodated.

Working during pregnancy

Unless your work involves heavy physical labour, or you work in an environment where there are harmful chemicals or fumes (*see p.23*), there is no reason why you should not continue working well into pregnancy. The length of time that you will work depends on your physical fitness, the sort of job you are doing and your reason for working. One benefit of working is that it encourages everyone around you to view pregnancy as normal. As well as that, your job gives you a feeling of stability and security during a time when you are undergoing physical and psychological changes.

There's no hard and fast rule about when to give up work – it depends on the nature of the work you do and how physically taxing it is. Between 32 and 36 weeks is a good time to stop as it's around then that the greatest workload is thrown on your heart, and other vital organs like the lungs, kidneys and liver; there's a great deal of physical stress on your spine, joints and muscles too. It's a time when you shouldn't be asking your body to do anything except rest if you're tired. This is difficult in a job, even a sedentary one.

Whatever your job, you will have to make adjustments to your daily routine. In later pregnancy, you will lose some of your agility, and working long hours and having late nights will leave you exhausted. You will find yourself falling asleep and having lapses in concentration. As far as your household chores are concerned, change your priorities. Your health and that of your unborn baby are far more important now than keeping a spotless house.

Being a working mother

Some women are happy to deal with pregnancy as a short interruption to their work, remaining in their posts until just before going into labour, then having the baby and returning to work in the shortest time possible. They avoid the emotional dilemma of whether or not to breast or bottle-feed the baby and opt for the latter. Other women would be unhappy with this decision. They want to stay with their baby; anything that takes them away from their child is painful.

Women with strong maternal instincts will be concerned with not only depriving their babies of affection, but also with the sacrifices that they are making themselves. They want to enjoy their children's presence and company much of the time, and, especially while their children are young, find it distressing to leave them even for a few hours.

Nonetheless, mothers continue to work for many different reasons, which include economic necessity, the desire to be independent and self-reliant, boredom with the routine of home life, and the absolute personal need to work. As women become more able to shape their own lives, more mothers are working, and of these more and more do so simply because they enjoy it. They feel that their work greatly enriches their lives and this in itself will help to enrich their family life.

In the past, many women thought it was their duty to ignore their own desires and serve the family (this attitude was often encouraged); now most women feel very strongly about having the right to take their own wishes into consideration and to make the decision to work if they want to, even if it may create complications in the family.

Your partner's feelings should also be considered along with your own. It can lead only to unhappiness and resentment if you decide to return to work but your partner is reluctant for you to do so. If you have reason to believe that he feels this way, you must bring matters out into the open. A frank discussion with him may lead to a suitable compromise and a happy solution to your working future.

Working in pregnancy
Continuing work as a theatre wardrobe mistress during her pregnancy provides this woman with stability at a time of emotional change.

When to return to work

If you decide that you are going to return to work after your baby is born, you might want to go back under different conditions. Discuss this with your employer during your pregnancy.

There may be provision for part-time employment in your work or a phased return that allows you to be, in effect, a part-time worker for a time after your baby's birth. You might like to investigate job-sharing or setting up on your own in some freelance activity, which might enable you to work from home. Now is the time to think about these alternatives and plan for them.

In figuring out when you are going to restart work, you must be fair to yourself. It takes about nine months for your metabolism to return to normal after a pregnancy; parts of your body recover more quickly than others. If you menstruate three months after giving birth, this is a good sign that your ovaries are getting back to their normal cyclical routine, but not all your hormone glands will be in step with them.

Your muscles, ligaments and joints become more flexible and elastic to accommodate your pregnant shape and weight and need time to regain their tone and strength. Vital organs like the heart, kidneys and lungs, and your blood, gradually adjust to coping with you alone and not you plus the baby.

Babies and parents

A good system of childcare will be a priority and you'll have to put quite a lot of time and effort into selecting one that suits your needs. If you feel reluctant or guilty about entrusting your baby to someone else, and fear that you might be left out of your child's affections, be reassured as I was (even though only in retrospect) by an interesting study carried out in the last few years. When I was a working mother with young babies, I didn't know that this research was going on and trusted my own instinct. What I felt was that my children would know me as their mother by the biological semaphore that I sent out and that they picked up. I felt certain in my own mind, despite the presence of very loving nannies, that my children could never mistake a nanny for me, their mother. I found it difficult to pin down how they would make the distinction. I thought possibly that it would be through body smell, and until they were about 18 months I made sure that they had opportunities to feel and smell my skin at feeding times and during nuzzling play.

Put your feet up
If you work right through your pregnancy, accept your condition and the stresses and strains pregnancy puts on your body. Sit down to work if you can and put your feet up whenever possible.

ADVANTAGES AND DISADVANTAGES OF BEING A WORKING MOTHER

Advantages

- Increased independence.
- Financial rewards – the chance to raise the standard of living of your family.
- Career fulfilment – the chance to use whatever training and qualifications you may have.
- More intense interaction with your child when you are at home.
- Intellectual need to work – you may feel bored and lonely at home.
- Ability to maintain a high profile in your chosen field of work.

Disadvantages

- You may feel a sense of guilt and inadequacy because you feel you are neglecting your child.
- Isolation from the community.
- Extreme tiredness because you will be juggling two jobs at once.
- Greater stress from dual responsibilities and the need to be constantly planning ahead.
- Resentment of the other full-time mothers in your community.
- Difficulty and concerns about finding and keeping good childcare.

What the research showed was that babies have an even keener intelligence for singling out their parents from all other human beings than I thought. The crucial factor for babies is the loving, interested attention that only parents can give, and a baby sorts this out from all the other stimuli. The most staggering aspect of this research is that babies need less than an hour a day of caring parental interest to thrive. The length of time spent without their parents counts far less than the quality of the time spent with them. Love isn't measured in time; love is what you put into time, no matter how short.

Dual role

Having to invest most of your free time in your family can be hard for a working mother. There's no denying that you are doing two jobs. Sometimes this is not too difficult. If you have an office job, you may have the energy to spare when you get home for bathtimes, play, story reading and sympathetic listening. However, a physical job or any job that involves caring or communication, means that during your working day you will be expending much of the sort of energy that you need for your children in the evening.

I firmly believe that a child, especially of pre-school age, has the right to expect and receive his parents' attention when they are home from work. The price of this is high. Instead of dropping into a chair or soaking in a bath when you return home, you'll have to pick up the baby and do everything else one-handed until he's asleep. When you finally fall asleep, ten to one your night will be disturbed. You don't just have to be generous of spirit, you have to be sacrificial too. There are advantages and disadvantages to being a working mother (*see above*); the best option for you is whatever makes you happiest.

Be prepared, however, for feelings of guilt and inadequacy, but so long as you and your partner are happy, you can be sure that your child will do equally well whether you stay at home or go to work.

3 Pregnancy calendar

Knowing about the changes that happen during pregnancy helps you to be more aware of your body and your needs. This month-by-month calendar summarizes what will happen. However, every pregnancy is different, so don't be alarmed if you haven't experienced certain changes by the date given here. Each month there's usually something else you need think about, such as booking antenatal classes. These are pointed out at the relevant time in the calendar but covered in more detail in later chapters.

Becoming pregnant

Signs of pregnancy

If you're planning a pregnancy and miss your period, you may suspect that you're pregnant. You may not notice any other changes apart from the missed period at first, but an increase in hormonal activity will confirm your pregnancy with one or more of the following physical signs:

- Feeling of nausea at any time.
- Change in taste: perhaps you will suddenly not be able to tolerate alcohol or coffee.
- A preference for certain foods, sometimes close to a craving.
- A metallic taste in your mouth.
- Changes in your breasts; they may feel tender and tingly.
- A need to urinate more frequently.
- Tiredness at any time of the day; you may even feel faint or dizzy too.
- Increase in normal vaginal discharge.
- Your emotions swing unpredictably.

Duration of pregnancy

Pregnancy lasts 266 days from the moment the egg is fertilized. Actual fertilization is usually difficult to pinpoint precisely. When estimating how pregnant you are, day one of your pregnancy is taken from the first day of your last menstrual period (LMP) and not the day of fertilization. If you have an average 28-day cycle, fertilization is counted as having taken place around day 14 and not day one of your pregnancy because ovulation usually takes place about 14 days before your period. The pregnancy timescale is thus 266 days plus 14 days – that is, 40 weeks. However, this is only a guide. The average normal pregnancy can last anything from 38 to 42 weeks.

Your developing baby
Understanding the changes that are taking place during your pregnancy and what you should do will help prepare you for the birth of your child.

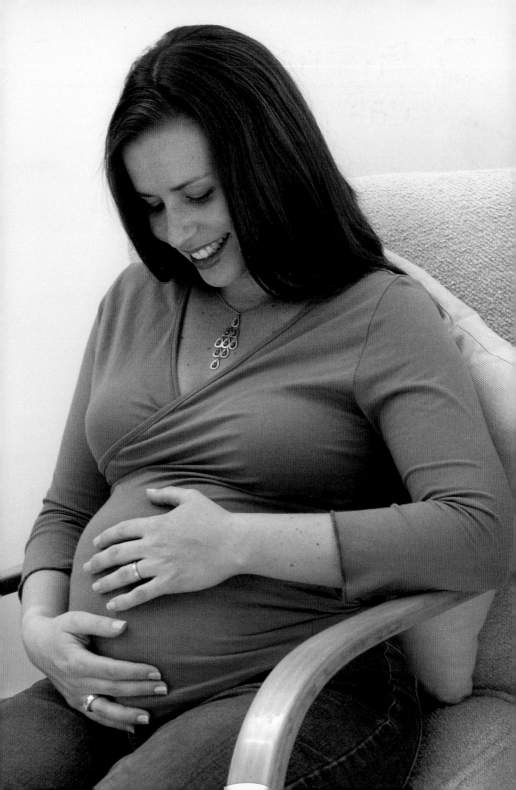

Weeks 6-10

By this stage of your pregnancy the uterus, which is usually the size and shape of a small pear, has become swollen and slightly enlarged, although it cannot yet be felt above the pubic bone. Visit your doctor to confirm the pregnancy and talk about the type of birth you'd like *(Chapter 4)*. You can also arrange your antenatal care, where and how to book in *(Chapter 5)*, although booking may not be done until between ten and 12 weeks.

Confirming your pregnancy

- The pregnancy hormone human chorionic gonadotrophin (hCG) can be detected in tiny amounts in urine. Home kits, available from chemists and larger supermarkets, are 99 per cent accurate and can confirm a pregnancy within a few days of your missed period. Another option is to go to your doctor or a family planning clinic for a test.
- A blood test could reveal the pregnancy hormones within a few days of you missing a period.

Tests in pregnancy

Your doctor will talk to you about screening tests such as blood tests, and ultrasound scans that are available to all pregnant women. You may also be offered diagnostic tests such as amniocentesis or CVS *(see pp.77–79)* if indicated because of your age or your personal or family history.

Take care

Your baby is most vulnerable in these first weeks, so you need to take precautions:

- Discuss any regular medication you may be taking before you try to conceive or as soon as you think you may be pregnant.
- Stop smoking and drinking alcohol.
- Find out if your work conditions are hazardous to your baby *(see p.23)*.
- If possible, check for rubella immunity before you conceive *(see p.14)*.
- Keep high standards of hygiene with pets to avoid toxoplasmosis infection.

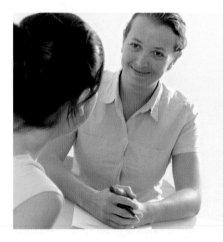

Antenatal care
At your first antenatal session, your booking-in appointment, the midwife will take a detailed medical history.

BABY'S DEVELOPMENT

The embryo, which can now be called a fetus, meaning "young one", has all the developing internal organs in place and is about the size of a small strawberry. The fetus is moving around a lot, although you cannot feel these movements yet, nor will you for a few weeks.

The fetus has a face with a nose, mouth and tongue

The heart and other internal organs are now established

Baby's appearance at eight weeks
Length: 25mm (1in)
Weight: 3g ($^1/_{100}$oz)

There's a metallic taste in your mouth and you may feel nauseous

Your breasts may tingle and feel heavy

Changes to your body
Your breasts may be feeling tender and heavier and you may experience nausea in the morning or at any time of the day. Your emotions may be unpredictable because of hormone fluctuations and you may feel very tired, which can make other symptoms feel more severe.

You need to empty your bladder frequently

Week 12

By this time, complaints such as morning sickness and frequent urination should have eased. You may notice a gain in weight for the first time. The amount of blood in your body increases steadily from now on so your heart and lungs have to work harder. Kidneys increase their work too. You may suffer some constipation as the bowel slows down. Keep up your normal fitness routine after checking with your doctor. Book a dental check-up.

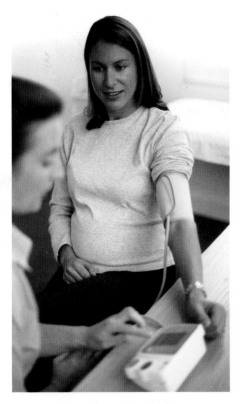

Blood pressure
Your blood pressure will be measured at every antenatal appointment. Regular checks mean that any change can be quickly noted.

Antenatal care

- You'll attend your first antenatal clinic if you haven't already (*see p.72*). During your pregnancy, you're entitled to paid leave to attend antenatal clinics and classes, so let your employer have details.
- You may be given a scan to check your dates and nuchal translucency (*see p.77*).
- This is a good time to decide on your course of antenatal classes. They provide lots of information and help you prepare for the birth. You'll also meet other parents whose babies are due around the same time as yours.
- The midwife or health visitor can tell you about local classes held either through the health centre or privately (*see Useful addresses p.242*). Private classes are usually smaller, less formal and may be in the tutor's home. They often specialize in antenatal exercises and techniques for managing labour with relaxation and breathing techniques (*see p.142*).
- If you have had problems with an incompetent cervix before (*see p.155*), a suture will be inserted at 12–14 weeks under a general anaesthetic.

BABY'S DEVELOPMENT

The eyes are completely formed and the baby's fingers and toes are developing, though they are still joined by webs of skin. Most of the internal organs are now working. The baby's movements are becoming stronger because his muscles are developing.

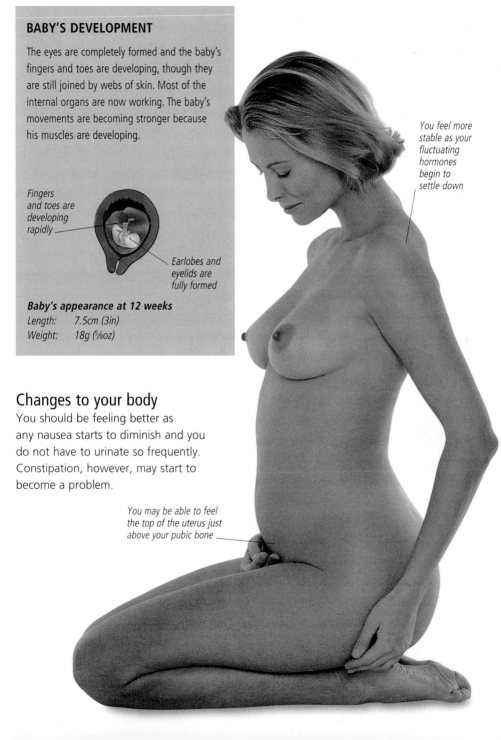

Fingers and toes are developing rapidly

Earlobes and eyelids are fully formed

Baby's appearance at 12 weeks
Length: 7.5cm (3in)
Weight: 18g (⅝oz)

Changes to your body

You should be feeling better as any nausea starts to diminish and you do not have to urinate so frequently. Constipation, however, may start to become a problem.

You feel more stable as your fluctuating hormones begin to settle down

You may be able to feel the top of the uterus just above your pubic bone

Week 16

You will start to feel better and more energetic. You will probably be noticeably pregnant now. Your muscles and ligaments begin to slacken and your waistline disappears. Choose your food carefully; your appetite will increase as you feel better and weight gain can be rapid. Start wearing comfortable unrestricting clothes (*see p.133*). If you haven't done so already, go out and buy a good bra with adequate support (*see p.135*).

Medical tests

- A screening blood test may be offered at 15 to 18 weeks to determine your risk of having a baby with Down's syndrome or spina bifida. Substances checked in this blood test are a protein produced by the liver called alpha-fetoprotein (AFP), oestriol and human chorionic gonadotrophin (hCG).
- Levels of AFP are usually low so if the test reveals that they are higher than normal it could indicate that you are carrying a baby with a neural tube defect. However, raised levels can also be caused by a twin pregnancy or by the pregnancy being further advanced than previously thought. Further tests will be offered before a definite diagnosis can be made.

Your baby's heartbeat
You may have an ultrasound scan between weeks 18 and 22. The sonographer will check your baby's size, her organs and her heartbeat.

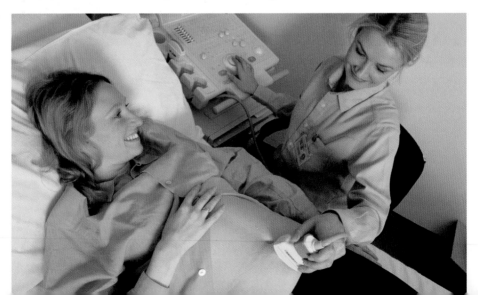

BABY'S DEVELOPMENT

The baby is now fully formed – she even has distinctive fingerprints. As the tiny bones inside her ears harden, the baby can hear sounds, for example, her mother's voice. Her movements become more vigorous and fine hair, known as lanugo, appears all over her body.

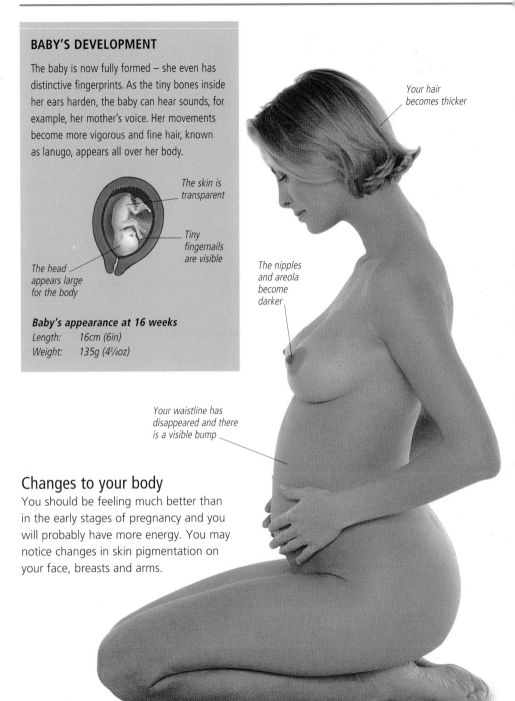

Your hair becomes thicker

The skin is transparent

Tiny fingernails are visible

The head appears large for the body

The nipples and areola become darker

Baby's appearance at 16 weeks
Length: *16cm (6in)*
Weight: *135g (4¾oz)*

Your waistline has disappeared and there is a visible bump

Changes to your body

You should be feeling much better than in the early stages of pregnancy and you will probably have more energy. You may notice changes in skin pigmentation on your face, breasts and arms.

Week 20

By now you can feel your baby's movements as light, butterfly-like ripples. You'll probably have an ultrasound scan between weeks 18 and 22, to check your baby's growth. It will also confirm if there is more than one baby. You should receive your maternity certificate (Form MAT B1) from your doctor or midwife. This entitles you to apply for statutory maternity pay or a weekly maternity allowance (*see p.247*).

Mixed feelings

It's normal for you and your partner to have mixed feelings about becoming parents. As you get nearer the birth your anxieties may increase as you question whether you're ready for parenthood and if it's likely to change your lifestyle and your relationship. By far the best course of action is to talk all these worries over. Another perspective is always valuable and may help you develop coping strategies.

Antenatal exercises

Exercise helps build strong muscles in preparation for labour so it's a good idea to plan an exercise programme at this time if you haven't already. At your antenatal classes, which continue throughout pregnancy, you'll be taught a number of exercises. You'll learn how to clench your pelvic floor muscles (*see p.122*) and increase your strength and flexibility in

preparation for labour. You can also exercise by yourself. Swimming is excellent for general fitness and you're supported in the water as you do some of your antenatal exercises (*see Chapter 10*). Always check with your doctor before starting any new exercise.

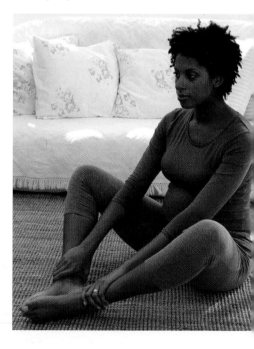

Fitting exercise into your day
Many exercises that are good when you're pregnant can be done at the same time as something else. Try tailor sitting while you're watching television.

BABY'S DEVELOPMENT

The genital organs can now be seen clearly
with ultrasound. The baby's teeth are forming
and, as his muscles develop, he's beginning to
move more vigorously. He'll move in response
to pressure on the mother's abdomen.

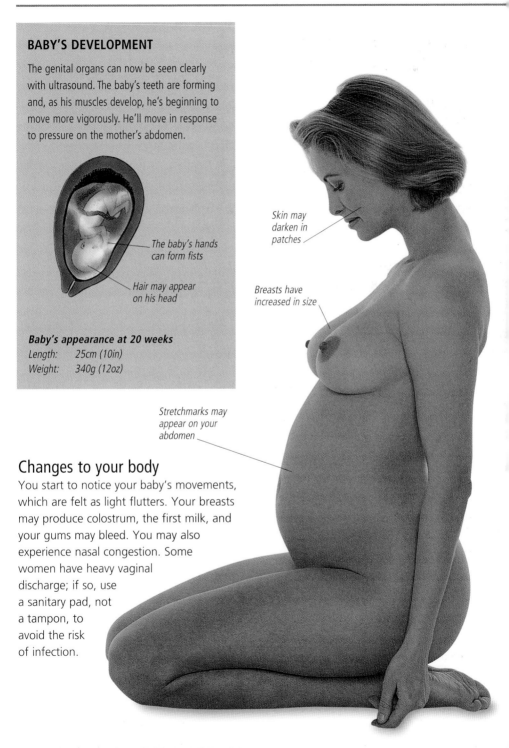

*The baby's hands
can form fists*

*Hair may appear
on his head*

*Skin may
darken in
patches*

*Breasts have
increased in size*

*Stretchmarks may
appear on your
abdomen*

Baby's appearance at 20 weeks
Length: 25cm (10in)
Weight: 340g (12oz)

Changes to your body

You start to notice your baby's movements,
which are felt as light flutters. Your breasts
may produce colostrum, the first milk, and
your gums may bleed. You may also
experience nasal congestion. Some
women have heavy vaginal
discharge; if so, use
a sanitary pad, not
a tampon, to
avoid the risk
of infection.

Week 24

Your greatest rate of weight gain takes place about now; your feet will start to feel the strain and you should watch your posture (*see p.118*). Ensure that your shoes are comfortable and rest with your feet up when possible. Your increased fluid levels may make you feel hot and sweaty and your face may be flushed because of increased blood circulation. If your baby was born now, she could survive with care in a neonatal intensive care unit.

Weight gain

You need to gain weight during pregnancy. Gone are the days when weight was watched obsessively and expectant mothers were admonished if they gained too much. Between weeks 24 and 32 there is usually the most rapid weight gain of pregnancy, but if you feel that you are gaining too much, this is the time to show some restraint or to increase your walking or swimming to use up any excess calories.

However, now is not the time to try to diet – wait until after the baby is born. Instead, eat a variety of nutritious and fresh foods.

Look after yourself
By now your heart and lungs are doing 50 per cent more work so take good care of yourself.

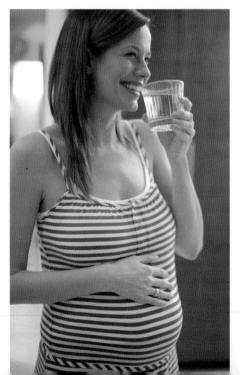

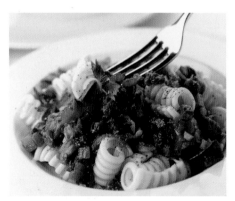

Eating in pregnancy
Try to eat a good variety of different foods in pregnancy. Choose fresh, unprocessed foods whenever possible.

BABY'S DEVELOPMENT

Creases start to appear on the baby's palms and fingertips and she can suck her thumb. She can also hiccup. The baby's patterns of sleeping and activity seem random, but unfortunately she may be most active when you're trying to sleep. The nostrils open and she is making breathing motions.

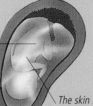

The body is now more in proportion to the head

The skin has lost its translucent quality

Baby's appearance at 24 weeks
Length: 33cm (13in)
Weight: 570g (1¼lb)

Your face may look puffy because of water retention

Increased circulation may cause you to sweat more

The bump is enlarging rapidly as the baby increases in size

Changes to your body

By now you are visibly pregnant and need to wear loose-fitting clothes. You may feel hot and sweaty because of your increased blood supply. Some women experience rib pain because the baby is pressing upwards against the ribcage.

Week 28

Tell your employer in writing when you plan to stop work; when the baby is due; and when you intend to return to work. Your antenatal checks may now be every two to three weeks. If born now, your baby has a more than 50 per cent chance of survival if cared for in a special care baby unit. A second blood test is usually done at 28 weeks to exclude anaemia, to check for blood group (rhesus) antibodies and to screen for diabetes.

Pregnancy complaints

Approach any minor discomforts of pregnancy sensibly *(see Chapter 13)* and be assured they will disappear after the birth. If indigestion troubles you, eat little and often and avoid problem foods. If you suffer from cramps, keep up your calcium intake with dairy products. Painless Braxton Hicks contractions may start to become noticeable *(see p.95)*.

You should be getting plenty of rest and sleep. This is not always easy as your size, the baby's movements and any digestion problems can make sleep almost impossible.

During the last months you may need to buy some loose tops, shirts and leggings to supplement your pregnancy clothing, or you could try borrowing clothes from your partner. For special occasions you may want to buy some maternity wear. Maternity dresses are usually longer in the front to allow for the bump. Wear low-heeled comfortable shoes.

Comfortable position
It may be hard to get comfortable. Use pillows to wedge yourself into relaxed positions at night and when you rest in the day.

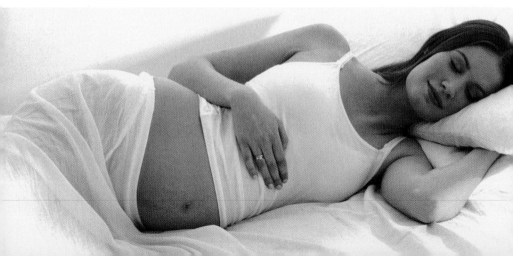

BABY'S DEVELOPMENT

Fat is building up under the baby's skin and he is coated in a waxy substance called vernix, which protects the skin so that it doesn't get soggy in the amniotic fluid. His eyes are open and he can see.

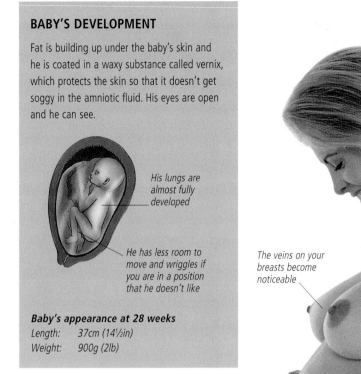

His lungs are almost fully developed

He has less room to move and wriggles if you are in a position that he doesn't like

The veins on your breasts become noticeable

Baby's appearance at 28 weeks
Length: 37cm (14½in)
Weight: 900g (2lb)

The womb has risen halfway between your navel and breastbone

Changes to your body

As you become bigger, you may notice stretchmarks on your stomach or thighs. Some women experience lower back pain, which is caused by the enlarging abdomen and loosening of the pelvic joints. As the uterus expands, you may suffer from mild heartburn or indigestion.

Week 32

If you exert yourself too much you will feel exhausted and breathless. You are probably looking forward to stopping work and should try to rest during the day if possible. Take things easy, especially if you aren't sleeping well. Parentcraft/antenatal classes will begin soon and you can prepare yourself by gathering all the necessary items for the birth (*see p.166*) and perhaps go shopping for the baby too.

Good posture

Stresses and strains are put on all your joints and ligaments during pregnancy. The change in your centre of gravity as the uterus enlarges can affect your posture and if you don't concentrate and think about your body when you pick things up and carry heavy bags, for example, you could suffer from unnecessary back pain.

Tiredness

If you find yourself lying awake, practise relaxation techniques. Hot-water bottles help soothe ribcage or pelvic pain. If you wake because you need to urinate, rock gently backwards and forwards while emptying your bladder. This helps to empty it more thoroughly, and should increase the interval before the next time.

Sex during pregnancy

In late pregnancy sex becomes difficult because of your size, so you may need to find more comfortable positions (*see p.105*) or other ways of loving. Massage not only soothes aches and pains but can be a positive way of showing affection.

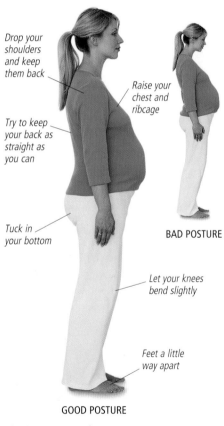

Drop your shoulders and keep them back

Raise your chest and ribcage

Try to keep your back as straight as you can

Tuck in your bottom

BAD POSTURE

Let your knees bend slightly

Feet a little way apart

GOOD POSTURE

The importance of posture
For good posture the head and spine are aligned; the shoulders are dropped and relaxed. With poor posture, the bulge at the front causes your back to arch.

BABY'S DEVELOPMENT

Most babies will have turned head downwards (cephalic position) in preparation for birth. If she was born now, the baby would have at least an 80 per cent chance of survival because her lungs have developed. The placenta has now reached maturity.

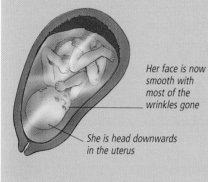

Her face is now smooth with most of the wrinkles gone

She is head downwards in the uterus

Baby's appearance at 32 weeks
Length: 40.5cm (16in)
Weight: 1.6kg (3½lb)

Your uterus starts to contract in practice for labour

Changes to your body

Your lower ribcage may feel sore and you may need to urinate more often as the uterus expands, putting pressure on your internal organs and diaphragm. Your navel will look flattened and a dark line (linea nigra) may be visible down the middle of your abdomen.

Week 36

Plan your life carefully now and get others to do all the running around. Strong Braxton Hicks contractions may make you believe you are in labour (*see p.95*). Take the opportunity to practise your breathing techniques. Antenatal clinics will be at least fortnightly until delivery. If this is your first baby, the head will "engage" (drop into the pelvic cavity); this eases breathing problems but pain may be felt in the pelvic region.

Breastfeeding bras

Your breasts won't enlarge any more until the milk comes in shortly after the birth. If you plan to breastfeed, now is the time to buy at least two front-opening nursing bras.

Wearing an ordinary pregnancy bra, measure yourself with a tape measure, noting both the chest and cup sizes. If you like, you can ask the shop assistant to measure you, or if you are not sure which sort of bra is suitable, ask for advice. If colostrum is secreted, you can wear breast pads to prevent stains on your clothing.

Preparation for birth

The nesting instinct becomes strong in the last trimester. You will probably have stopped work now so will have time to buy clothes for the baby and prepare a room with a cot, changing mat, nappies and other necessary items (*see Chapter 15*). This nesting instinct can lead to bursts of activity, but try not to overdo it. You will need all your strength later for labour and birth. Around this time you also need to prepare clothes and other items you will need for your delivery (*see pp.166–167*).

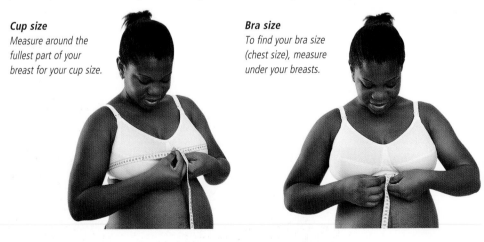

Cup size
Measure around the fullest part of your breast for your cup size.

Bra size
To find your bra size (chest size), measure under your breasts.

BABY'S DEVELOPMENT

The baby is steadily putting on weight. He may now have lots of hair and his fingernails have grown to reach the end of his fingers. The irises of his eyes are blue.

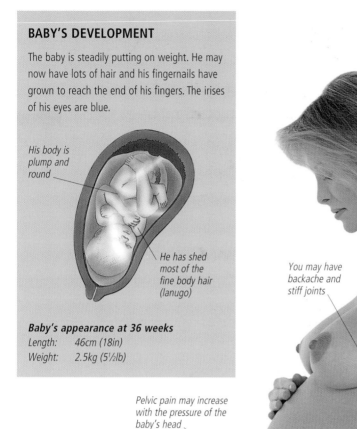

His body is plump and round

He has shed most of the fine body hair (lanugo)

Baby's appearance at 36 weeks
Length: *46cm (18in)*
Weight: *2.5kg (5½lb)*

Pelvic pain may increase with the pressure of the baby's head

You may have backache and stiff joints

Changes to your body

As the baby's head drops into your pelvic cavity, irritating digestive problems and feelings of breathlessness should lessen. It may be more difficult for you to get a good night's sleep as your large abdomen can make it difficult to find a comfortable position.

Week 40

The expected date of delivery is near and you may be anxious when it passes. Don't worry – only five per cent of babies arrive on the due date. You'll be feeling very heavy and tired; all your movements will be an effort, and as the baby is lying deep in your pelvis, you may have pain in the groin and pins and needles down your legs. The baby's movements decrease in force (although not in frequency) because there's less space for her.

Signs of labour

Braxton Hicks contractions may be so strong that you think you are in labour. If in doubt, call the hospital or your midwife. True contractions are more regular than Braxton Hicks. Labour isn't always signalled by a definite sign (*see p.171*). You may have a "show" of blood-tinged mucus that has blocked the cervix during pregnancy. This show may happen up to two weeks before the onset of true labour, but is a sign that it is not far off. Other signs are a leakage of amniotic fluid and contractions occurring at regular intervals.

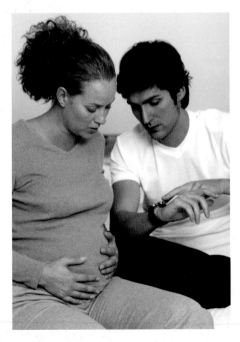

Timing contractions

Time contractions over an hour to find out whether this is true labour. Keep a check on both the length of contractions and the interval between each one. They should become stronger, more frequent and last for 30 to 60 seconds. Sometimes contractions start and then fade away. When your contractions are coming every 15 minutes, are about a minute long, and don't die away when you move around, telephone your midwife and let her know how things are going.

When to go to hospital
Plan to go to hospital when your contractions are coming at five minutes apart or less, if your waters break or if you are bleeding.

BABY'S DEVELOPMENT

The baby is full size and, if it is a boy, the testicles will usually have descended. If this is your first baby, the head will have already engaged in the pelvis.

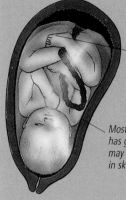

Her fingernails are long and she may have scratched herself

Most of the vernix has gone, but some may still be present in skin folds

Your skin feels tight and itchy

Baby's appearance at 40 weeks
Length: 51cm (20in)
Weight: 3.4kg (7½lb)

Changes to your body

You are feeling very tired and all your movements take a lot of extra effort. Your lower abdomen feels very heavy and your skin is tight and uncomfortable. You may want to clean the house in readiness for the birth, but try to conserve your energy.

Your cervix is softening in preparation for labour

You may get pins and needles in your legs and feet

4 Choices in childbirth

Most women are aware that there are choices to be made in childbirth and, given a normal pregnancy, they can exercise many options. In most parts of the UK, doctors and midwives form flexible teams that work towards satisfying a woman's preferences. You should feel that the birth of your child is an experience over which you have control and that you're free to enjoy. Hospitals welcome your partner or someone else close to you as a birth attendant. Home births are also becoming more common with the advent of the team midwife scheme. A doctor no longer needs to be present at a home birth, but the woman must be taken to hospital if complications occur.

Organizing yourself

In theory, there's no reason why you shouldn't have exactly the kind of birth you want, but it's up to you and your partner to make sure you're able to take an assertive, informed part in the way your labour and delivery will be handled.

Some women are disappointed by their experience of childbirth; not the birth itself but the way it's conducted or the way they're treated. If you're going to have the kind of birth you want, first, you need to be clear in stating your desires. Second, you have to be aware of your options. The way you can achieve this is by reading, asking questions, writing to various associations for information and guidance (see pp.242–246), and never accepting anything unless you feel entirely happy about it. Third, you also need to communicate what you want. Set things

out on paper in a logical way so that they are clear in your own mind. Ask your partner or a good friend to come along for moral support when you're seeing your doctor or midwife.

One aim of this chapter is to make it easy for you to plan the kind of childbirth you would like after assessing your own emotional and physical needs. Another aim is to give you the confidence to discuss with doctors and midwives on equal terms the options available and to state your preferences. Most hospital notes have a page for you to record your birth plan so that your wishes are available for all your attendants to see.

A family event
If you have your baby at home the whole family will feel involved with the new addition from the start.

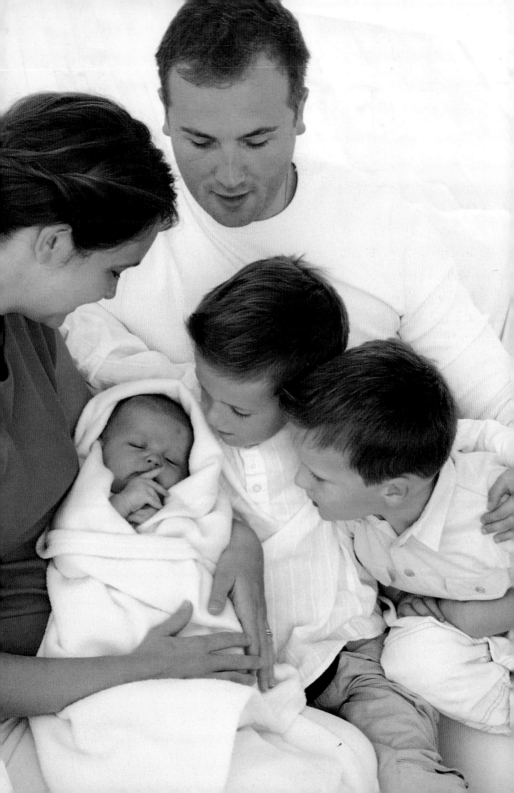

Getting information

Spend some time finding out where and how you are going to have the baby. One of the first things to do is to talk to your doctor. He or she will give you information about what is available and the various people that you might get in touch with. Your doctor will also tell you the kind of birth he or she recommends and you'll be able to assess if you're going to get on easily or if there may be conflict. This will help you to make a decision. At the same time contact your midwife. More and more women are opting for midwife-supervised births; and while it's always advisable to work with your doctor, most recognize now that a normal birth can be handled perfectly safely by a trained midwife. Your midwife will give you the addresses of the various associations to write to.

WHERE TO HAVE YOUR BABY

The two important elements in your choice are whether you want a medically managed or a natural childbirth and whether you want to have your baby at home or in hospital.

There are people who passionately advocate hospital high-technology births, who say that this is the only way to ensure that mother and baby will be well looked after, especially if an emergency occurs. At the other extreme, there are the natural childbirth advocates who are equally vehement in support of their methods. Some women feel that only in a hospital will they find the security they need. Other women wish to be surrounded by hearth and home when they give birth to their baby. Think about the following options.

Consultant maternity unit

This is obstetrician-based care within a general hospital. Most antenatal care is done in the community; however, women who may have complications attend the antenatal clinic at the hospital. In this case you may well be seen by different doctors and midwives at each visit, though now many hospitals have introduced team midwives. Most centres across the country now have birthing pools and other facilities so a woman can have the labour she prefers. For first-time mothers the support of other mothers and hospital staff during the first days is an advantage, although a busy hospital may not be restful for some.

The emphasis in a hospital maternity unit will be on helping you to have a normal birth. However, it's here that you're more likely to experience so-called "high-tech" obstetric procedures, which are available if necessary.

Team community midwife scheme

A community midwife from a local team looks after you antenatally in partnership with your own family doctor. When you go into labour, your regular midwife, or one who is on call at the time, will take you to hospital and deliver you there. You can go home with your midwife within six hours of the birth if all is going well, and you're unlikely to be in hospital more than 48 hours. This scheme isn't available in all areas.

At home

At one time medical opinion was almost 100 per cent of the view that a hospital delivery was safer than a home birth. However, studies have shown that women are much more relaxed at home and it has been proved that it's at least as safe to give birth at home as in hospital for a healthy mother and her baby. Most midwives will agree to a home birth if they feel it's safe for the mother.

Home birth

There are advantages to giving birth to your baby at home if your pregnancy is straightforward. You'll avoid exhausting travel to hospital when you're already in labour, and you'll have the same midwife throughout labour and birth. Starting off breast-feeding is nearly always more successful in the home environment. The other important factor is that you lead the way in managing your labour and birth; others support you.

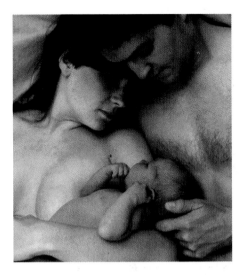

Familiar surroundings
After a home birth, you'll all feel more relaxed as you're in your own familiar surroundings.

Family group
By staying at home you'll avoid all the unhappiness that can be caused by family separation, particularly if you have other children. In addition, everyone can benefit from the emotional and physical bonding immediately after the birth.

Mobility
This is now recognized as being positively helpful during labour. Most women find it easier to cope with contractions if they are able to change position at will; it also helps the uterus to work better and keeps the oxygen to the baby topped up. Although hospitals encourage mobility, many women prefer to have the freedom and privacy of moving about in their own home.

Confidence
You'll probably feel confident and relaxed because you're in a familiar place. This is a great advantage, as emotional well-being does affect the function of the uterus. You'll also avoid the possibility of cross-infection from the medical staff and other mothers and babies in hospital. Being at home will avoid many of the aspects of hospital care that you may find distasteful. Their absence will be a bonus.

Organizing a home birth
Home births are now organized through the community midwife. Once you've made a request for a home birth, the community midwife will need to perform a risk assessment at your home. Unless there are very good reasons for you not to have a home birth, you shouldn't encounter any obstacles. Midwives are obliged to support a woman in her choice of birth.

If you have difficulty finding a midwife to attend a home birth, contact the Director of Midwifery in your area, or get in touch with one of the associations working towards improving maternity services, such as AIMS (*see p.245*).

Hospital birth

For some women the decision to have a hospital birth is made for them because of their physical condition or their obstetric history. However, if you do need or want a hospital confinement, before you decide on a particular hospital, there are many questions that you may want to ask. Use this checklist to help you:

- Can my partner or friend stay with me during labour and delivery?
- If I need a Caesarean section, can my partner or a friend be with me?
- May I walk around during labour if everything is okay?
- May I choose the position in which I can give birth?
- Do women have their waters broken as a routine?
- What percentage of women do you induce in this hospital?
- How many women have continuous electronic fetal monitoring?
- What percentage of women have an episiotomy or a forceps delivery in this hospital?
- Can I arrange to have no drugs for pain relief in this hospital?
- When a Caesarean birth is planned how many women have epidural anaesthesia and how many have general anaesthesia?
- Can I have as much time as I want to cuddle my baby after delivery if everything is okay?
- If I have a Caesarean section can I and/or the father hold the baby afterwards?
- Can I use aromatherapy oils during labour for massage?
- Is there flexible visiting time?
- Is it possible to arrange a six-, 12- or 24-hour discharge?

WHY A HOSPITAL DELIVERY?

For some women there are good reasons for having a hospital birth:

- If your medical history includes conditions such as heart or kidney disease, high blood pressure, tuberculosis, asthma, diabetes, serious anaemia, obesity or epilepsy.
- If your previous deliveries have included a stillbirth, a transverse or oblique lie (that is if the baby is lying sideways in the pelvis), premature labour before the 37th week, placental insufficiency where the placenta failed to nourish the baby adequately, or a retained placenta. (A previous vaginal breech delivery is not a contraindication as long as the current baby is in a head down position.)
- If the following obstetric reasons apply in your case: true postmaturity (see p.199); you have pre-eclampsia; you're carrying twins or higher multiples; your baby is in the breech or transverse position; you have experienced bleeding from the vagina late in pregnancy; you have placenta praevia; there is excessive water around the baby; you're a Rhesus-negative mother and tests have shown that there are sufficient antibodies in your blood to harm the baby; you have scarring of the uterus from previous Caesarean sections or you're over 35 years old and you're expecting your first baby (although this is no longer necessarily a reason for special attention in hospital provided you're healthy – see p.14).

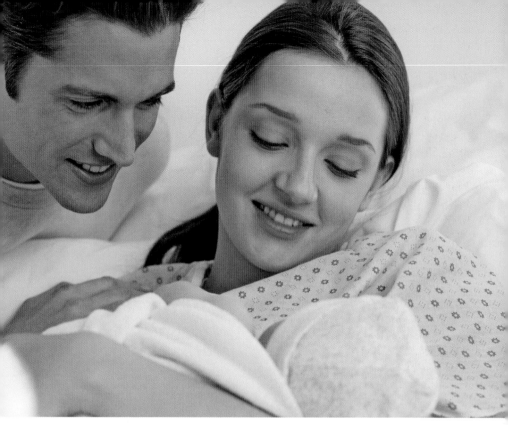

How long?

Your hospital stay can be as short as six hours and this is becoming increasingly normal in busy maternity units. A fairly standard stay is 24 hours or less, and even after a Caesarean you may be discharged after 48 hours provided the incision is healing and the baby is healthy. However, it is your right to discharge yourself from hospital, on your own responsibility, at any time. If you have adequate support and help and there are no complications with either you or your baby, there is no reason why you should not go home.

Your birth partner

Your partner should be closely involved in the pregnancy and birth, and he's the natural choice for a birth assistant. His

Helping you through labour
Your partner or a friend will be able to stay with you in hospital to encourage you throughout your labour and the delivery of your baby.

involvement is crucial, not only as support for you but also for cementing the bonds with the baby from the moment of birth. He can be the most loving and supportive "midwife". His involvement from the beginning of pregnancy will improve your communication in preparation for the birth, and during labour your partner is the person who gives you most attention. The medical staff are there to support the two of you. However, your birth assistant doesn't have to be your partner. You may prefer to have a relative or close friend with you instead or even as well.

The midwife

A midwife-supervised pregnancy and labour guarantees continuity of care, a factor that is missing from many hospital pregnancies. Whenever you attend the antenatal clinic you will see one of the team midwives so you can get to know them all during your pregnancy, and one of the team will attend you during the birth.

The obstetrician

Some women feel cheated and nervous, even second class, if they don't have an obstetrician as well as a midwife present at their delivery. Despite the fact that they expect nothing to go wrong, they would simply be happier in the hands of a specialist.

There is yet another group of women for whom the hospital setting makes childbirth the event they expect it to be.

Under normal hospital circumstances, obstetricians usually only attend difficult births and emergencies, so you can expect to pay quite a substantial amount for private attendance. Private health care in the UK does not usually cover antenatal care, or delivery except for Caesarean section. Obstetricians are very busy, and on your day of delivery the doctor you want may not be available; you may not see the same doctor at each antenatal visit.

If you want to go privately, obtain a list of practitioners from the Royal College of Obstetrics and Gynaecology (*see p.242*).

The natural childbirth movement

As obstetric medicine became more sophisticated, childbirth gradually came to be seen as a medical condition – something to be overseen by doctors – instead of the natural, straightforward process that it really is. However, from the 1960s onwards there has been a movement by women (helped and supported by midwives) to reclaim natural childbirth. This means giving birth without fear, without unnecessary medical intervention and in a calm atmosphere.

Several methods were propounded with slightly differing emphases, some of which centred on the mother, others on the baby, and still others on both. But the net result was a gradual and welcome changing of attitudes so that in the majority of hospitals the best points of

the different approaches have been adopted and developed. Originally, however, there was a pure form of each method.

Grantly Dick-Read

In his book *Childbirth Without Fear*, first published in the 1940s, Dr Grantly Dick-Read brought the principles of natural childbirth to public attention. His philosophy was to try to lessen and hopefully eliminate fear and tension, and the pain that resulted from these emotions, through proper education and emotional support. The Grantly Dick-Read method taught women how to cope with tension but lay strong emphasis on the fact that knowledge allays fear and prevents tension, which in turn controls pain. To help this, Grantly Dick-Read developed courses that included breathing control exercises and relaxation of muscles (*see p.142*), information on what to expect in a normal situation, and what women can do to help themselves. He also taught mothers how to look for support in the form of guidance, reassurance and sympathy. He also laid great store on preparation for parenthood and childbirth itself.

Psychoprophylaxis

This involves training in breathing methods as a preparation for labour. The techniques were pioneered in Russia and introduced in the West by Dr Fernand Lamaze. The Lamaze method is by far the most popular in the United States and is the basis for the teaching of the National Childbirth Trust in Britain. It encourages the woman to take responsibility for herself, to enter into partnership with her companions, friends and counsellors. It greatly values team work. The woman must prepare her body throughout pregnancy with special exercises and she has to train her mind to respond automatically to each type of contraction she will feel in labour. Her partner acts as "coach" and provides emotional support. He is expected to attend the course with the expectant mother and co-operate with her at home on the conditioning exercises, and he coaches, coaxes and comforts her throughout labour and delivery.

The Leboyer philosophy

This relies on several basic precepts and relates more to the baby than the mother and her progress throughout labour. Dr Frederick Leboyer in his book *Birth Without Violence* states that the newborn baby feels everything, reflecting all the emotions surrounding it – anger, anxiety, impatience and so on – and that the baby is extremely sensitive through its skin, ears and eyes. For that reason he believes that all stimulation to the baby should be minimized with low lights, few sounds, little handling, and with immersion in water at body heat so that the baby's entry into the world is as similar to its life in the womb as possible.

This teaching is in fact not entirely in line with the physiology of what occurs at the moment of birth for the baby. It is contact with air at a temperature different from body temperature that makes the baby take its first gulp of air to start the initial crucial function of the lungs and causes the baby's blood circulation to change from a fetal one to a mature one. It is also simply not true to say that a baby's hearing is so sensitive that it is disturbed by noises around it. The sound of the uterine vessels within the womb are akin to a loud vacuum cleaner. Leboyer also believes that the mother is an "enemy and a monster" to the child, driving it and crushing it within the birth passage. He likens her to a torturer. Many women quite reasonably object to this view as it minimizes, even diminishes, the role of the mother.

Dr Leboyer believes that the baby should not be touched by foreign materials but by human skin. The ideal place for the baby is to be laid face down on the mother's abdomen and covered by her arms. It has been proven by experiment, not Leboyer's, that this is far more efficient in preventing the baby from losing heat than overhead heaters. Research has shown that a baby is able to clear mucus from its respiratory passages far more efficiently when lying face down on its mother's stomach than with a suction tube.

Leboyer suggests that the curtains and blinds in the delivery room are drawn and the lights are dimmed. Some medical authorities object to this as they say it is not possible to assess the baby's condition in a dim light.

Few centres practise the pure Leboyer method, but many hospitals and community midwives practise Leboyer-based birth. It seemed to me on first reading Leboyer that all he had done was to formalize what midwives had been doing, in principle, for years. Hospitals were slower to adopt Leboyer because research has shown that the babies appear to receive no extra benefit compared to others, though many "Leboyer mothers" may feel they do.

Dr Michel Odent

A French doctor named Michel Odent has advocated placing the mother in an environment that is cosy and home-like, giving her complete freedom to act as she wishes and encouraging her to reach a new level of animal consciousness where she forgets her inhibitions and returns to a rather primitive biological state. Dr Odent believes that the high levels of endorphins, the body's natural narcotics, should be allowed to have full rein in the mother's body. He logically argues that if a woman is given pain-killers and analgesics, her endorphins are cut off, thus depriving her of the benefit of natural pain relief.

Dr Odent's clinic in Pithiviers in France, where he pioneered his natural childbirth techniques, became a centre for those who wished to change opinions and practices in childbirth. Dr Odent believes that during labour there should be music, soft furnishings, and a relaxed atmosphere. A woman who goes into labour should be allowed to sit, walk, stand, eat and drink, and do whatever she wants. Women should not be interfered with in any way and can take up whatever position is most comfortable at any stage of the labour. Left to their own devices many women take up a position on all fours, which seems to help the pain. Later on in labour many stand up or semi-squat so that the force of gravity can help them, a natural thing to do, which most primitive tribes practise. Odent encourages the supported squatting position where the woman's partner, stands behind her, takes her weight underneath her armpits and upper arms and allows her to bend her knees and place her weight on her partner's arm.

Dr Odent believes that birthing pools, which he now uses for many home water births, should be primarily viewed as a means of pain relief. The birth itself does not need to be underwater, though Dr Odent is quite happy to deliver the baby into the water of the bath. There seems to be no proof that an underwater birth is dangerous to the baby so long as the head is lifted out of the water immediately.

Dr Odent's methods have always had low rates of episiotomy, forceps and Caesarean section. The supported squat position is the one that prevents severe perineal tears during delivery. Because the mother has been in an upright position when the baby emerges she remains sitting upright with the cord still intact and the baby in her lap. The baby smells the mother's skin and it's thought that this is important to the baby in establishing breast-feeding. Within a few seconds most mothers instinctively lift their baby to the breast. No partner needs to be told to encircle the mother and the baby; each will do what comes naturally to them.

Yoga-based methods

This is not just for women who already practise yoga. During childbirth a woman should concentrate her awareness on being totally at one with what is happening to her. Through yogic methods she is able to control her awareness according to her capacity and tolerance so at some times she is able to distract herself from the contractions and at others be totally involved in them. She may use meditation and chanting with the support of yoga groups' spiritual participation. Practitioners in the yogic methods believe that a woman can handle childbirth in a mature and serene way. Yogic childbirth education helps in the belief that a woman has the ability to create or destroy her own pain and joy during birth.

Nursing and medical procedures

One of the most welcome outcomes of the natural childbirth movement has been the shift in emphasis back to the mother and her needs in hospital births. Practices that were once routine such as enemas and shaving pubic hair are no longer performed, and mothers are not confined to bed; in fact even epidurals allow some mobility. Midwives and hospital staff constantly review procedures and guidelines. They have accepted wholeheartedly the findings of much research from around the world that has proved the efficacy of mobility during labour.

An excellent study done in Latin America has shown that in a group of mothers having their first baby, the length

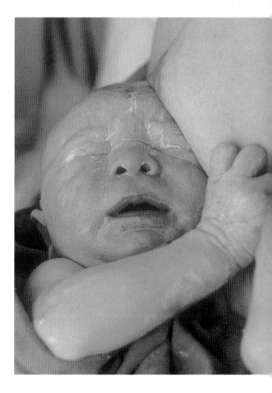

First contact with your baby
When a newborn baby is held against his mother's body, he immediately learns to recognize her smell and may start to suck.

of labour in those who were allowed to move around as they wanted to was only two-thirds that of the women who were confined to bed. When all mothers were considered, the mobile group were 25 per cent quicker in producing their babies than those who did not move around.

The study also found that 95 per cent of mothers who are left to themselves prefer to be upright and are more comfortable when upright. When mothers spend time in different positions in labour they report less pain and greater comfort when sitting, standing, kneeling or squatting.

The study concluded that in normal spontaneous labour, women who are allowed to assume a vertical position generally have an easier, shorter labour, with less discomfort and pain. In the light of all this, no doctor or midwife would now deny women who are having normal labours the right to choose the position or positions that they find most comfortable during the first and second stages of labour, since this is likely to be the most advantageous position for them in terms of their pelvic shape and the position of the baby. Lying on the back for delivery is now positively discouraged for the reasons that are given below.

Positions for delivery

Before the end of the seventeenth century when labour rooms were solely the province of women, no one considered that the normal behaviour of a woman in childbirth should be interfered with. She was allowed to move about as she wanted, take up any position that she felt was comfortable, eat and drink as she wished and assume her chosen position for delivering the baby. Then doctors invaded the delivery room and at that time all doctors were men. A doctor at the French royal court proposed that women should lie on their backs in preference to using upright positions and birthing stools to make vaginal examinations and obstetric manoeuvres easier, not because it might benefit the mother or the baby.

It is natural for a woman to take up a semi-vertical position for delivery of the baby, not just because it's comfortable but because it is mechanically most efficient. When a woman is upright, the uterine contractions are aiming downwards, pushing the baby out towards the floor. When a woman pushes, she strains

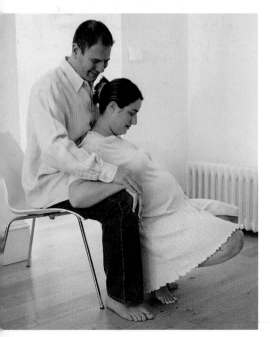

Keeping upright
More and more women now prefer to give birth in a vertical or semi-vertical position. The force of gravity helps to push the baby out.

downwards in the same direction and most importantly the force of gravity helps the birth of the baby.

When a woman lies on her back, the uterine contractions push the baby into the delivery bed and not down the birth canal so the added advantage of the force of gravity is lost. The result is that the recumbent woman has to push her baby up and against the force of gravity. This not only prolongs labour but makes it more likely that complications may occur (*see box, below right*).

In most hospital birth units, women are allowed to give birth in the position that they find most comfortable. If a ventouse or forceps delivery is necessary your legs may need to be put in stirrups, so that the doctor is able to use the instruments most effectively and follow the contours of your pelvis while delivering the baby. This will mean less trauma for the mother. However, even in these circumstances you should still be propped up with pillows, not lying completely flat on your back.

Food and drink
During labour the stomach seems to close down, and any food eaten during this time may be vomited up. For this reason it is a good idea to have something light and easily digestible to eat very early in labour while you're still at home to give you reserves of energy. Take glucose tablets into the delivery room with you in case you have a sudden demand for energy.

Most hospitals let women eat or drink during labour if they wish, but those at high risk of needing an emergency general anaesthetic will be advised not to. However, I don't believe that this is a good enough reason to withhold food from all women – it should only be the policy for those who are definitely at risk of needing a surgical procedure.

Most women in labour don't want to eat but most do require fluids, particularly as labour advances and fluids are lost through sweating, so water should be given, in my opinion, whenever it is requested. If a mother is denied water, so starts to become dehydrated during labour, an intravenous drip may have to be set up to administer glucose solution directly to the mother's bloodstream, bypassing the stomach and thereby increasing the medical intervention in her labour.

The delivery room
In most hospitals nowadays you will go through labour and deliver your baby in the same room. The only time you are likely to be moved is if you have to have an emergency Caesarean because most delivery rooms are not big enough to accommodate all the equipment safely.

DISADVANTAGES OF LYING ON YOUR BACK FOR DELIVERY
If you lie on your back:
- Your blood pressure may drop, thus reducing the amount of blood and oxygen to the baby.
- Pain is greater in this position than if you can be vertical.
- There's a greater need for an episiotomy.
- There's an increased chance of your having a forceps delivery.
- It inhibits spontaneous delivery of the placenta.
- There is a greater possibility of low back strain in this position.

At your antenatal clinic ask about the delivery rooms. Most hospital-based antenatal classes will include a tour of the delivery suite and postnatal wards; try to do this so you know what to expect. Most delivery rooms now have soft lighting, pictures on the walls and pleasant, homely soft furnishings. There will be a bed (not an old-fashioned delivery table), but you may also be able to use a mat on the floor or a beanbag for back support. Some more progressive units make birthing

pools available as an aid to pain relief. If there is no pool in the hospital you are going to, it may be possible to hire one.

You may also be able to use aromatherapy during labour: to perfume the birthing pool, in massage oil and on your pillow. Ask what is available in your hospital and what you can bring with you to make your labour comfortable. You'll be able to deliver almost exactly as if you're at home but with medical facilities on tap should either you or your baby need them.

Choosing how to feed

The most important aspect of infant feeding is nourishing the infant. Most babies thrive whether they are breast- or bottle-fed. Given that as a basis (and in your worst moments remind yourself of this as your overriding priority), think about the other considerations.

In order to make a choice and exercise an option you have to be aware of the pros and cons of breast- and bottle-feeding or a combination of both. You must bear in mind your own preferences because feeding will be most successful if you're happy with the method you have chosen. And you must also think about what is best for your baby. Although bottle-feeding is convenient, there's little doubt that as far as the baby's well-being is concerned, breast-feeding is superior.

Advantages of breast-feeding

A good reason for breast-feeding is that it's the natural thing to do. Most women have an instinctive urge to breast-feed, and

there are very few women who are not physically equipped to breast-feed. No matter how small their breasts, they will be able to produce enough milk to feed and sustain the baby. Even women whose nipples are inverted can, with early diagnosis, breast-feed their babies (*see p.93*). Other advantages include:

• It's normal for a mother to feel proud that her baby is being fed on food that she provides and it's natural to crave the physical nearness and pleasure and to know that you're helping to develop a close relationship with your child.

• Breast-fed babies are less liable to illness than bottle-fed ones. There are fewer cases of gastroenteritis, chest infection and measles. All the mother's antibodies to bacterial and viral infections are present in the colostrum, the first milk made by the breasts that is present in the breasts from the fifth month of pregnancy. In the first few days of life, therefore, when the baby is taking only the high-protein colostrum, she is living under the umbrella of her mother's antibodies. They have a protective effect in the intestine but also, as they're absorbed straight into the baby's system unchanged, they form an important part of the baby's own protection against infections. Take the example of a mother who has antibodies to poliomyelitis in her own body. Because those antibodies appear in her colostrum, it's not possible to infect her baby with the poliomyelitis virus while she's being wholly breast-fed. Any antibodies in the baby's gut will kill the virus before it can do any harm.

- Human milk is antibacterial because it contains substances that destroy bacteria. Even though these substances are present in formula milk, a bottle-fed baby is not protected in the same way because the antibodies are inactivated when the cow's milk is heated.
- Human breast-milk is the best source of food for a human baby; it has just the right amount of minerals and proteins. Cow's milk, which is for calves, has a

higher percentage of protein and a high content of casein, which is the least digestible part of it and is passed out in the stool in the form of curds.
- Human milk contains just the right amount of sodium (salt) for a newborn baby. This is important because the immature kidneys of the infant are unable to deal with high levels of sodium in the blood. Cow's milk contains more sodium than human milk.
- While human milk and cow's milk contain the same amount of fat, the droplets in human milk are smaller and more digestible. Breast-milk fat is high in polyunsaturates and low in cholesterol, and it may therefore protect against heart disease in later life.
- Breast-milk contains more sugar (lactose) than cow's milk and the mineral and vitamin content is different.
- Breast-feeding is good for your figure. Research has shown that a woman loses most of the fat she's accumulated during

Lying down to breast-feed
You can lay your baby next to you while you lie down so she can feed from your lower breast. This is also a good way to breast-feed after a Caesarean operation.

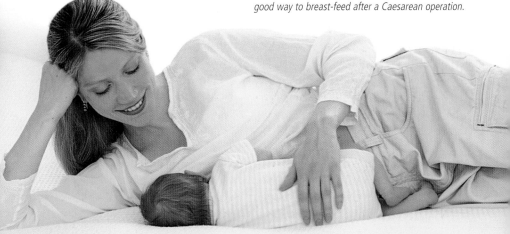

pregnancy if she breast-feeds. If you don't feed your baby yourself, you'll probably have more difficulty returning to your pre-pregnancy weight.

• It's a common fallacy that the breasts lose their shape and firmness through breast-feeding. This is not so. The changes that occur in the breasts are a consequence of becoming pregnant, not of producing milk or feeding your baby.

• Breast-feeding also has the advantage that it releases the hormone oxytocin, which encourages the uterus to shrink to its non-pregnant size.

• Breast-feeding is convenient. Milk is always available at any time of the day or night, it doesn't have to be made up, there's no expensive equipment to buy and keep sterile, and it's free.

• Bonding occurs between mother and baby quite automatically if you breast-feed. When a baby is at the breast, her face is close to her mother's face – about 20–25cm (8–10in) – and even a newborn baby can focus at this distance (see p.212). The act of making eye contact and smiling at your baby as she sucks, helps to create a strong physical and emotional bond between mother and baby that they will build on for the rest of their lives.

Overcoming disadvantages

One of the often quoted disadvantages of breast-feeding is that it curtails social activity. This need not necessarily be so. During the early weeks babies are very portable and you can take your baby with you when you go out. Although feeding in public places can still cause raised eyebrows, it's easy to feed discreetly, and many bigger shops, restaurants, train terminals and airports now have designated baby-feeding areas.

If you don't want to take your baby out with you, you can express sufficient milk with a breast pump (see p.236) to serve the baby's needs while you're away from her. You can bottle your own breast-milk in sterile bottles and store them in the fridge or freezer and your babysitter can give the bottle to your baby later on your behalf. Remember, even if you only feed your baby for two weeks, that's better than not breast-feeding at all and it will give your baby a flying start in life. Incidentally, one of the advantages of expressing some of your milk into bottles is that your partner can be involved with feeding too.

Bottle-feeding

As there are no real arguments against breast-feeding, it is also true to say that there are no arguments in favour of bottle-feeding. However, for some women, breast-feeding may not be a feasible or workable alternative, in which case bottle-feeding will be your choice. If it is, don't feel that your child is getting second best.

• Babies thrive and are perfectly happy being bottle-fed, and always remember that your baby needs your love and care more than she needs your breast-milk. Bottle-feeding, love and attention are an excellent option for any baby.

• There will be certain mothers who don't have any option but to bottle-feed. These are women who may be taking drugs in the long term for a medical condition, such as epilepsy, which needs barbiturates to keep it under control, or chronic depression for which antidepressants are prescribed. You may become seriously ill and need admission to hospital. If physically you're not in a fit state to breast-feed, then you should not. If you have to take any medicines regularly, discuss with your doctor whether they are passed on to your baby in breast-milk and what the possible effects will be on breast-feeding and your baby. Quite often it's possible for nursing mothers to change to safer drugs.

- Some disabled babies, or babies with physical abnormalities such as cleft palate or deformity of the jaw and mouth, may not be able to suck successfully and will have to be spoon- or bottle-fed.
- If you think your milk supply is inadequate and your baby is failing to thrive, consult your midwife or a breast-feeding counsellor before opting to bottle-feed. Your own nutrition and physical fitness do have a bearing on successful breast-feeding so you need to make sure you're getting a balanced diet (*see p.110*).
- Some women have a strong physical revulsion against breast-feeding and find it a chore. A woman who feels revulsion very strongly will be under stress when feeding, and this may interfere both with milk production and milk flow. If you feel that your baby is not getting enough milk, these negative messages will also reinforce your dislike of breast-feeding. If this happens to you, do try to talk over your feelings before the birth of your baby with a sympathetic friend or midwife and do involve your baby's father in the discussion.
- One of the main advantages of bottle-feeding is that your partner can be

equally involved in feeding your baby from the beginning, which allows him to create a close, nurturing bond with his baby early on.

- Bottle-feeding also means that you can work out a shared feeding schedule with your partner that gives you each enough time for rest, for unbroken sleep and for time off for yourselves.
- One of the questionable advantages of bottle-feeding is that babies sleep longer between feeds during the first weeks (although this is by no means always the case). This longer sleeping period could be because the casein content of cow's milk is higher than that of human milk and takes longer to digest.
- When you're bottle-feeding, you can see exactly how much milk your baby has taken at each feed, which some parents find reassuring.

PROBLEMS WITH BOTTLE-FEEDING

- The posset from a bottle-fed baby has an unpleasant smell, as do the stools.
- Some babies are allergic to the alien protein in cow's milk. There are substitutes for babies with allergies; nursing mothers in families with a history of eczema or asthma are advised to breast-feed or use these substitutes.
- The sterilization of bottle-feeding equipment and the careful preparation of feeds are time-consuming compared to the accessibility of breast-milk.
- Bottle-fed babies are more prone to gastric infections than breast-fed babies, who receive some protection from their mothers' milk.
- The cost of formula milk, bottles, teats and sterilizing equipment is substantial, whereas breast-milk is free and is always available.

5 Antenatal care

Good antenatal care is the key to healthy mothers, happy pregnancies and thriving babies and its importance can't be over-emphasized. It's now accepted by most doctors that the best way to improve the statistics on childbirth is through early and vigorous antenatal care. By talking to doctors and midwives at antenatal clinics, and to other mothers, you can find out more about pregnancy and birth, which should reassure you and make you feel more confident. Much of the antenatal care is routine, but at the clinic you can ask questions and explore the different circumstances in which you can have your baby so that you can plan for the kind of birth you want.

Going to the doctor

As soon as you suspect or know that you are pregnant, make an appointment to see your doctor. He or she will want to know the date of the first day of your last menstrual period (LMP) as it's from this day that the pregnancy is measured. Depending on how far your pregnancy is advanced, your doctor will perform some kind of pregnancy test – either a urine test (*see p.26*) or a blood test if you've missed at least one menstrual period. Your doctor may want to confirm the pregnancy even if you've already used a home kit yourself and know that you're pregnant.

The first visit to your doctor is important not just for confirmation of the pregnancy. It's at this meeting that you can discuss in general terms your options for the birth (*see pp.52–67*), so give the subject some thought before you go along

– for example, would you like a home or hospital birth. Your preferences may conflict with your doctor's desire to stick to routines and procedures that she's used to and is reluctant to change, particularly with regard to home births. It's helpful for your partner to accompany you to this first appointment so you can discuss these issues together and iron out any difficulties from the start.

If you're over 35 or you have some history of genetic disorders in the family, you may need to see an obstetrician about having chorionic villus sampling (*see p.77*). This procedure should be done between weeks ten to 12, so visit your doctor early to get a letter of referral.

Use your doctor as a source of information: ask for a list of recommended books to read and pamphlets to send off for. If your own doctor does not specialize in obstetrics, you may need to see another member of the practice, or you may be referred to a neighbouring practice where they undertake antenatal care and home birth if this is what you want.

The other option is to attend the local hospital or the hospital of your choice depending on your area. In which case you'll be looked after by the team of midwives and the medical staff at the hospital and not by your own doctor.

Antenatal clinics

After confirmation of the pregnancy your doctor will make arrangements for your antenatal care. This will depend upon the sort of birth you want. Most antenatal care is now undertaken at community antenatal clinics run by midwives, not at hospitals. You should only need to go to the hospital clinic for your first visit when you need to have a scan, blood tests and so on. You will only have to go to a hospital clinic more than once if there is a specific reason why you need to be examined by an obstetrician, such as high blood pressure, or if you have some underlying medical condition such as diabetes.

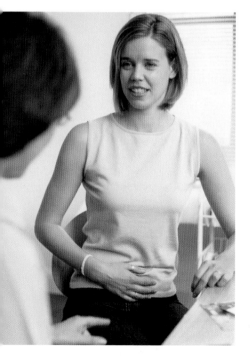

Antenatal clinic
This is your opportunity to ask questions about your pregnancy as well as for the midwife to assess you. You can also find out about antenatal exercise classes.

COPING AT THE CLINIC

These days, you shouldn't have to wait too long for your appointment at the hospital antenatal clinic. However, just in case there is a delay, try to make the best of your time there by preparing in the following ways:
- Take your partner or a friend along to chat to or a book or magazine to read.
- Take some water and a small snack such as some fruit with you as it may be difficult for you to get to the cafeteria.
- Make notes of all the questions you want to ask and note any worries even if you're not sure whether they're linked to your pregnancy.
- Try to get your other children cared for while you go to the clinic; it's hard to keep them entertained so they may get bored and make you feel stressed.

ROUTINE ANTENATAL TESTS

Test	Purpose	Significance
Height and weight 1st visit	To calculate your BMI (body mass index). If you're very overweight or underweight, you may need extra care. This also gives your midwife a benchmark figure in case of problems later.	Excessive weight gain can strain heart; sudden gain may indicate pre-eclampsia (see p.160).
Lungs, hair, eyes, teeth, nails 1st visit	To check on your general physical health.	You may need vitamin supplements or just dietary advice. Dental visits will be encouraged.
Legs and hands every visit	To look for varicose veins and any swelling (oedema) in the ankles, hands or fingers.	Cases of extreme puffiness can be a sign of pre-eclampsia (see p.160). Advice on what to do about varicose veins will be given (see p.152).
Urine (MSU) 1st visit	To test for kidney infection. Clean vulva with sterile pads, then pass urine into a sterile container. Let the first drops to go into the toilet and collect the mid-stream urine (MSU) only.	Existing underlying kidney infection can develop into a serious condition in pregnancy. You will be treated with antibiotics.
Urine Every visit	**1** Tests for protein in case your kidneys aren't coping well. **2** Tests for sugar; if sugar is found repeatedly, you may have diabetes.	**1** Protein in urine late in pregnancy may be a sign of pre-eclampsia (see p.160). Bed rest will probably be prescribed. **2** Pregnancy can unmask diabetes (see p.154), which must be stabilized. It may go after delivery only to return in later pregnancies.
Fetal heartbeat Every visit after week 14	To confirm that the fetus is alive and that the heart and heart rate are normal.	If the midwife listens to your baby's heart with a sonicaid (this monitors the fetal heart with ultrasound vibrations), the sound of the beat will be amplified so you can hear it too.

Test	Purpose	Significance
Abdominal palpation Every visit after 24 weeks	To assess the height of the fundus (the top of the uterus – see p.74), and the size and position of the fetus.	Gives a guide to the size of the baby. Palpation by a midwife after 34 weeks will indicate the lie of the fetus and whether the baby is in the breech position (see p.202).
Blood pressure Every visit	This is the measurement of the pressure at which the heart pumps blood through your body. The reading has two numbers: the first is the systolic pressure, when the heart contracts, pushes out blood and "beats"; the second is the diastolic pressure, the resting pressure between heartbeats. A normal BP is 120/70.	High blood pressure (hypertension) can indicate a number of problems, including pre-eclampsia (see p.160). Constant checks mean it can be kept under control if it suddenly rises, for example above 140/90. May mean bed rest in hospital if it rises. Any rise in the lower or diastolic figure is cause for concern.
Blood tests 1st visit: tests 1–8 16 week visit: test 4 28 week visit: tests 1–3	1 To find your major blood group: A, B, AB or O. 2 To find your Rhesus blood group. 3 To find your haemoglobin level (repeated test). This is a measure of the oxygen-carrying substances in your red blood cells. Normal levels, measured in gm., are between 12 and 14gm. 4 Alpha-fetoprotein (AFP) levels – a special test at 16 weeks (see p.75). 5 To detect the presence of rubella (German measles) antibodies. 6 VDRL, Kahn or Wasserman tests for the presence of syphilis. 7 To detect or confirm sickle-cell disease and thalassaemia, conditions mainly found in dark-skinned people and those from the Mediterranean. 8 To check whether the mother is HIV positive (done by consent).	1 Blood group needed in case of an emergency transfusion. 2 In case of Rhesus incompatibility (see p.160). 3 During pregnancy your haemoglobin level may drop, because you have more circulating blood. If it falls below 10gm, treatment for anaemia (see p.154) will be given in the form of iron and folic acid supplements that raise the haemoglobin level so that more oxygen can be carried to the baby. 4 See p.75. 5 To find out if you have rubella immunity (see p.14); if not, you will be warned to avoid contact with rubella. 6 If you unknowingly have this sexually transmitted infection, it must be treated before week 20 of your pregnancy; after this time it can be passed to the baby. 7 Can affect the baby and the pregnancy. If either condition is found and you were not already aware of it, you will be given folic acid supplements. 8 Treatment will be given to decrease the chance of infection in the baby.

The first visit

The purpose of your first visit to the antenatal clinic at around 12 weeks is to give information to the staff so that they can judge whether or not your pregnancy and delivery is likely to be normal. If you're planning a home delivery, you'll be asked about the social and domestic side of your life to assess whether the circumstances are suitable for home delivery.

The staff will also run tests to check your health (see pp.70–71); for instance, taking your blood pressure, collecting a sample of your blood and testing your urine. The results will be available at your next visit.

Ask questions, too. It's important for you to gain confidence in your pregnancy by expressing any concerns. It isn't essential now at the first visit, but it's as well to discuss your preferences for pain relief during the labour, whether you want an early discharge, and what course of action you want if the baby is overdue. Your file and notes will be made available to you. At the end of the visit you may be given iron tablets (see p.113) and you can ask to

YOUR ANTENATAL FILE

At the initial interview you'll be asked some or all of the following questions about your relevant medical and past obstetric history:

• Your name, age, race, date and place of birth, marital status, as well as the name of your next of kin.
• Your childhood illnesses, and whether or not you have ever been in hospital or had any serious disease or any surgical operations.
• If any illnesses run in your family or your partner's family.
• Whether there are twins in either family.
• Whether you used contraceptives, if so what sort and when you stopped.
• Your menstrual history: when your periods first started, how long your average cycle is, how many days you bleed and the date of the first day of your last menstrual period.
• Whether you have any pregnancy symptoms and what your general state of health is like.
• The births of any other children you may have, or any miscarriages.
• Whether you're taking any prescription medicines or suffer from any allergies.
• What work you and your partner do and whether you're still working.

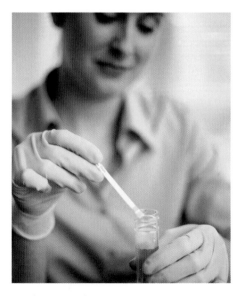

Testing your urine
At every antenatal visit you will be asked to supply a sample of your mid-stream urine. Routine tests will be done on the sample immediately and the results will be marked in your notes.

see a dietitian if you need information about diet and nutrition. You'll probably attend the antenatal clinic every four to six weeks up to 36 weeks, and thereafter every two to three weeks. Check-ups are more flexible than they used to be, and their frequency will depend on your health and the health of your baby.

When you enrol at an antenatal clinic you'll be told about the antenatal classes and will be given details of where they're held and at what time.

The medical staff

- A midwife is trained in the care of women with normal pregnancies and the delivery of their babies. If all goes well a midwife will deliver your baby whether at home or in hospital. Midwives also work in the community and once you return home after delivery, you will be visited by a midwife every day until ten days after the birth of your baby.

- Your family doctor may be responsible for part of your antenatal care. He or she may attend your delivery at home, although family doctors do not routinely attend home births; if all is well they're happy to leave it to the midwife.

- The obstetrician is the hospital doctor who specializes in pregnancy and birth. He or she heads the team of midwives, nurses and other doctors who provide your antenatal care and deliver your baby. The consultant obstetrician should usually be on hand in the hospital delivery unit to supervise and teach the junior doctors.

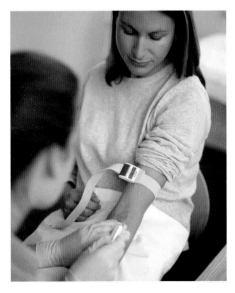

Taking a blood sample
A routine sample of your blood will be taken twice during pregnancy, and tested for specific problems and as a general check on your health. The first sample is sometimes also used to confirm the pregnancy.

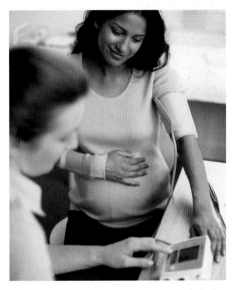

Taking your blood pressure
This is measured at every visit so that any change can be quickly brought under control. Raised blood pressure may be a sign of pre-eclampsia, so you'll be closely monitored by your doctor and midwife.

UNDERSTANDING YOUR HOSPITAL NOTES

At your first antenatal visit you'll be given your hospital notes. At every visit your doctor or midwife will record on them details of the routine tests and the progress of the pregnancy. Take your notes with you to every clinic. Keep them with you if you go out of your area – if you should need medical attention, all the information will be at hand. Most of the abbreviations are explained below.

NAD/nil/	Nothing abnormal discovered in urine	Height of	The height of the top of the uterus.
Alb	Albumin (protein found in urine)	fundus	The baby pushes this up as it grows
BP	Blood pressure		and often the height is used to
FH	Fetal heart		estimate the length of the
FHH/NH	Fetal heart heard or not heard		pregnancy. Some clinics measure
FMF	Fetal movements felt		the height of the fundus (from the
Ceph.	Cephalic, the baby is head down		top of the pubic bone to the top of
Vx	Vertex, the baby is head down		the uterus) in centimetres. This is
Br.	Breech, the baby is bottom down		usually roughly the same as the
LMP	Last menstrual period		pregnancy in weeks.
EDD/EDC	Estimated date of delivery or	Relation of	This is the brim of your pelvis.
	confinement	Presenting	The presenting part (PP) of the baby
Hb	Haemoglobin levels to check for	Part to brim	to the brim in the later stages of
	anaemia		your pregnancy will be the part in
Eng/E	Engaged, the baby's head has		your cervix ready to be born first.
	dropped into the pelvis ready for birth	Oed.	Oedema
NE	Not engaged	RSA	Right sacrum anterior – the most
Para O	Woman has no other children		common breech position
Para 1	Woman has one child	AFP	Alpha fetoprotein
Fe	Iron has been prescribed	CS	Caesarean section
TCA	To come again	H/T	Hypertension
PET	Pre-eclamptic toxaemia	MSU	Mid-stream urine sample
Long L	Longitudinal lie, the baby is parallel to your spine in the womb		

The lie of the baby
These abbreviations describe the way the baby is lying and refer to the position of the crown of the head (Occiput) in relation to your body – on the Right or Left, to the front (Anterior) or back (Posterior).

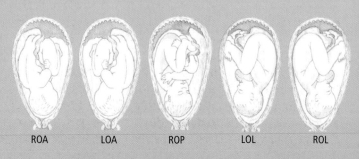

ROA   LOA   ROP   LOL   ROL

The older woman

Nowadays the age of the mother is much less important than her medical history, diet and lifestyle *(see p.12)*. However, if you're over 35, you may still be asked extra questions at your first antenatal appointment. Once all the questions are answered, any tests performed *(see below)*, and you're found to be generally fit and well, your care will be no different from that of younger women.

Parentcraft/antenatal classes

First-time parents can gain confidence and information from these classes. They should ideally cover an understanding of pregnancy and birth; techniques of relaxation and breathing to prepare for labour; and caring for a young baby. Hospital-run classes will help you understand the procedures in that hospital and you will be able to see the delivery suite and postnatal wards.

Special tests

There are a number of tests available to check for any potential physical or chromosomal abnormality in the fetus.

AFP screening

Alpha fetoprotein (AFP) is a substance found in the blood of a pregnant woman that varies in level throughout pregnancy. Between 16 and 18 weeks of pregnancy the blood AFP levels are usually low. If your blood is examined for AFP at this time, and the levels are raised, it could indicate that you are carrying a baby with a neural-tube defect such as spina bifida, or other abnormalities of brain development.

Raised AFP levels in the blood are not, however, conclusive evidence of neural tube defect. In addition, AFP levels may be raised with a twin pregnancy and may also rise as pregnancy progresses. If a blood test indicates raised levels, an ultrasound scan will be taken to check for twins or to confirm your dates in case the pregnancy is more advanced than you thought. A further blood test will then be taken. Only if all of these checks prove positive and if corroboration is needed will amniocentesis be contemplated because to be certain, alpha fetoprotein must also be found in abnormal quantities in the amniotic fluid. Minor neural tube defects such as a small hairy mole at the bottom of the spine are quite common.

Lower than normal levels of AFP indicate the risk of Down's syndrome; in this case amniocentesis will be offered.

Triple test

This is another maternal blood (serum) screening test, also known as the Bart's triple test, the Leeds test, the Biomark, or the Beta Triple. It also measures other hormones present in the woman's blood, such as oestriol and human chorionic gonadotrophin (hCG). The test is done between 15 and 18 weeks. The results can be assessed alongside your age to predict the chance of your baby suffering from Down's syndrome. If the chances seem high, amniocentesis will be offered.

Ultrasound scan

This works by giving a photographic picture that is formed by creating images from the echoes of sound waves bouncing off different parts of the body of different consistencies. Unlike X-rays, ultrasound can show soft tissue in detail and will give a very accurate picture of the fetus in the uterus. Ultrasound is very useful as a way of determining the age of the fetus, the position of the placenta and therefore your expected date of delivery. Any visible abnormalities will be picked up clearly by the scan technician.

The first scan is often given at around 11–13 weeks of pregnancy, to establish the age of the fetus, and for nuchal translucency (*see opposite*). A second scan given at 20–22 weeks will check that your baby is growing properly. The scan can take 20 minutes or more. You may have been asked beforehand not to pass urine and, if this scan is early in your pregnancy, to drink plenty of fluids so that your bladder is full, which helps your uterus be clearly visible to the technician. Wear loose clothes so you can easily lift them off your abdomen. Oil or jelly is spread onto your stomach and a

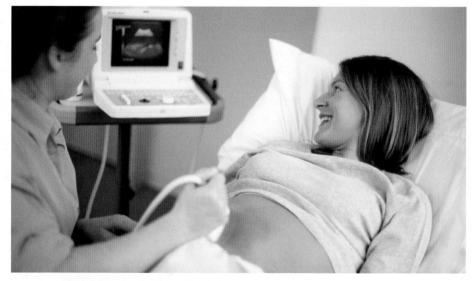

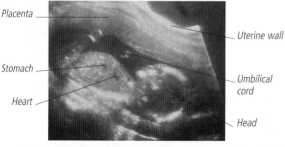

Placenta

Stomach

Heart

Uterine wall

Umbilical cord

Head

ULTRASOUND IMAGE OF BABY

The fetus in utero
It is very exciting to see a picture of your baby moving about in your womb. Ask the technician to point out the head, limbs and the baby's organs. The ultrasound procedure is painless but if you have a scan in the early part of your pregnancy you will need to have a full bladder. Don't worry about this; arrive early and drink several glasses of water.

transducer is passed over it, which sends back signals onto a black and white monitor. You will feel no pain, just a soft, oily, flowing sensation on your stomach.

Nuchal translucency scan

Also known as an NT test, this is a test used to assess the risk of Down's syndrome. A high-definition ultrasound scan can be carried out to measure the collection of fluid at the back of a baby's neck. All babies have some fluid, but a higher than normal reading can be an indication of an increased risk of Down's syndrome. A high reading does not necessarily mean there is a problem, but it would indicate the need for further tests, such as chorionic villus sampling or amniocentesis, to be done. The NT test should be carried out between weeks 11 and 14 of your pregnancy, and research studies have shown it to be about 75 per cent accurate. When combined with a blood test the accuracy rate rises to about 90 per cent.

Chorionic villus sampling

If you have a family history of genetic disorders or if you've had an affected baby previously, it is likely you will see the obstetrician early in pregnancy to discuss prenatal testing such as chorionic villus sampling (CVS), which is usually done when you're ten to 12 weeks pregnant.

The CVS test takes about 15–20 minutes. A small sample of the chorion (the outer tissue that surrounds the developing fetus and placenta) is taken and analysed. Using an ultrasound scan to guide the probe, a fine, hollow tube is inserted in the vagina or through the

abdominal wall and into the uterus. A few of the chorionic cells are sucked out; these cells are identical to those in the fetus. Analysis will show if the baby has a chromosomal abnormality.

Occasionally, CVS may lead to rupture of the amniotic sac, infection and bleeding. Even so, it only seems to increase the risk of miscarriage by one per cent. This test is performed earlier in pregnancy than amniocentesis and the results are available in about 10 days. CVS therefore gives the choice of an early termination, rather than having to wait longer for an amniocentesis.

USES OF ULTRASOUND

An ultrasound scan is used by medical staff to:
- Help determine the age of the fetus by taking measurements of the head and body. If the scan is done early in pregnancy, it will be accurate to within one week.
- Determine if you are carrying one baby, twins or more babies.
- Locate both the position of the placenta and its condition.
- Find out the exact position of the baby and placenta before an amniocentesis (*see p.78*).
- Pick up visible abnormalities of the baby such as brain or kidney conditions.
- Identify any fibroids in the mother that might hinder delivery.
- Measure the growth of the baby and if clinical examination suggests something is wrong, serial assessment – that is a number of scans over a period of time – can be performed. Growth restriction may be discovered and early delivery recommended.

Amniocentesis

Used to detect a range of chromosomal defects, amniocentesis is not a routine test. It may be carried out if you're over the age of 37, as the risk of chromosomal abnormalities increases with age; or if the obstetrician suspects some abnormality that cannot be detected by other tests. Although it is readily available, it is still a serious interference with your pregnancy. It involves taking a sample of the fluid surrounding the baby in the uterus. Any discarded cells floating in the amniotic fluid will give an accurate chromosome count for the baby and denote abnormal chromosomal structure.

Many women over 37 are concerned to see if their baby has any abnormalities. If you're worried, talk to your obstetrician.

Most obstetricians will agree to this test to give you peace of mind. They will also offer amniocentesis if you already have a child with an abnormality, or if there is a family history of abnormality. The sex of the baby can be determined by simply looking at some cells of the skin so you can find out if any gender-linked disorders might have been inherited. However, doctors will not do the test simply to find out the baby's sex. In cases of Rhesus incompatibility, the bilirubin content of the fluid is a good indicator as to whether the baby needs an intrauterine blood transfusion (*see p.160*).

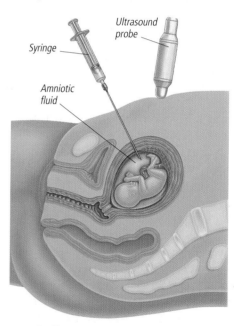

How the fluid is extracted
After an ultrasound scan to determine the position of the fetus and the placenta, a small area of the abdomen is numbed with local anaesthetic and a long hollow needle surmounted by a syringe is carefully inserted into the womb. About 15–20ml (½–¾fl oz) of fluid is then drawn out. The cells shed by the baby are separated from the amniotic fluid for analysis.

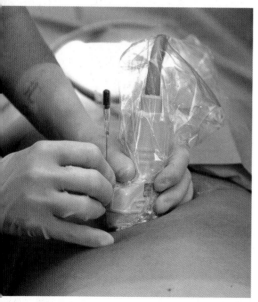

Having an amniocentesis
Amniotic fluid from around the baby is drawn off from the womb. The fluid is then analysed to provide a chromosome analysis of the baby.

How amniocentesis works

Amniotic fluid is swallowed by the fetus and passed out through its mouth or bladder; this fluid contains cells from the skin and other organs that provide clues under analysis to the baby's condition. Amniocentesis is the procedure to extract this fluid from the womb.

About 75 different genetic diseases can be diagnosed by amniocentesis. The test is done in hospital, generally not until 14–16 weeks after the last menstrual period; before then there is unlikely to be sufficient fluid in the amniotic sac and therefore not enough cells to analyze.

Risks of amniocentesis

With a skilled operator and the use of an ultrasonic scan to show the exact position of the placenta and the fetus, the risk of miscarriage is less than that with CVS (*see p.77*) – below one per cent in Britain, and 0.5 per cent in the United States.

When deciding to have amniocentesis you need first to weigh up the reasons for you being offered it against the risk of miscarriage. You also need to think about whether you're prepared to have your pregnancy terminated if the results give cause for concern.

Possibly the worst element of amniocentesis is the stress of waiting for the result, although this should be no more than three weeks. Many women talk about putting their pregnancies "on hold" at this time. Also your amniotic fluid may only be tested for a single abnormality, which means that a negative result may not reflect other possible problems. Ask your doctor for the results of all possible tests that could apply to you.

REASONS FOR AMNIOCENTESIS

- Amniocentesis will be offered if you're over 37, when the risk of chromosomal abnormalities increases greatly and you may be at risk of carrying a baby with Down's syndrome, for example (*see chart below*).
- The test can give parents the chance to decide whether they want to continue with the pregnancy if the test is positive. In some cases it may also allow for the early detection and treatment of a disorder while the fetus is still in the womb.

DOWN'S SYNDROME

This is the result of a chromosomal abnormality in the baby. In most cases an extra chromosome occurring before or immediately after fertilization gives the fetus 47 chromosomes in each cell instead of the normal 46 (*see p.18*). The exact cause is unknown, but maternal age is an important factor. The risk of having a baby with Down's syndrome rises sharply after the age of 35.

APPROXIMATE PROPORTION OF AFFECTED BABIES PER 1000 BIRTHS

20   25   30   35   40   45

WOMAN'S AGE

6 The growing baby

Pregnancy can be roughly divided into three parts, or trimesters, each lasting around 12 weeks. By the end of the first trimester, the fetus is recognizably human, although only 7.5cm (3in) long. The second trimester is a period of rapid growth, and during the third trimester the baby gets longer and starts to accumulate fat.

Life-support systems

The successful growth and development of your baby depends on a healthy placenta. The placenta is the organ that allows your baby to depend on you and your body functions for his health and well-being. It acts as a waste disposal unit and cleanses the baby's body of unwanted waste materials. It does so through its unique structure, which allows the intermingling of your blood with your baby's blood. It's useful to think of the mature placenta as a blood-filled space, bounded on each side by a maternal surface and a fetal surface.

Amniotic fluid

From week four or five, amniotic fluid fills the amniotic sac, formed by the bag of membranes enclosing the embryo. By week 12 the baby is swallowing the fluid, which is absorbed via his intestines into his bloodstream. From there it passes through the umbilical cord and the placenta into the mother. Early in the second trimester the fetus begins to use his own kidneys and to urinate. Excess vernix, nutrients and products necessary for the maturing of the baby's lungs are also in the amniotic sac.

WHAT AMNIOTIC FLUID DOES

- Supports the baby while he moves freely, thus helping him to exercise its muscles.
- Cushions the baby in the uterus.
- Exerts a constant outward pressure on the uterus so the baby has room to grow.
- Protects the baby's head during labour while assisting cervical dilatation.
- Maintains a constant temperature.
- Receives substances excreted by the baby in urine.

WHAT THE PLACENTA DOES

- Allows oxygen, nutrients and protective antibodies to be passed from mother to baby.
- Produces essential pregnancy hormones.
- Passes the baby's waste to the mother.

The membranes

These are two thin, papery sheets, the amnion and the chorion, which line the uterus and form the bag of waters inside which the baby develops.

Baby's life-support system

The amniotic space and the placenta make up the baby's life-support system. The amniotic space develops deep inside

the blastocyst, formed by the fertilized ovum and contains traces of cells that bear the sex of the embryo and the blueprint of its genetic make-up (*see p.19*). The space is surrounded by the membranes and it contains the amniotic fluid or "liquor". The placenta is joined to the baby by the umbilical cord. This cord is made up of three intertwined blood vessels. Two carry blood from the baby to the placenta for cleansing and purification. One carries oxygenated blood and nutrients to the baby. The cord is surrounded first by a jelly-like substance (Wharton's jelly) then by a membrane. The placenta itself is firmly rooted to the wall of the uterus.

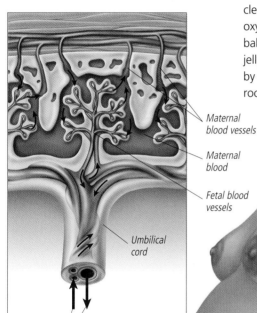

Maternal blood vessels

Maternal blood

Fetal blood vessels

Umbilical cord

Direction of blood flow to and from fetus

Fetal surface of placenta

Umbilical cord

Amniotic fluid

The placenta
The blood coming to the placenta's maternal surface carries oxygen plus nutrients for the baby, which are absorbed through the fetal surface. Blood from the baby carries away waste products including carbon dioxide.

First trimester

By the end of the first trimester, the systems of the fetus's body are already well developed, with many organs more or less complete. Nerves and muscles are working, and reflexes are becoming established. The heart pumps about 30 litres (52 pints) of blood through the circulatory system each day. Your baby can move spontaneously, although you're not aware of these movements.

Week 5

The embryo is quite easy to see with the naked eye. The spinal column is beginning to develop. The foundations of the brain and the spinal cord are appearing.
Length: 2mm (⅛in)

Week 6

The head begins to form, followed by the chest and abdomen. The immature heart is beating. Blood cells are circulating. Blood vessels are forming in the umbilical cord to

the placenta. There are small depressions where the eyes will develop and the beginnings of a mouth. The lower jaw is visible. There are arm and leg buds.
Length: 6mm (¼in)

Week 7

Indentations that will form the fingers and toes are visible. The intestines are almost completely formed. The lungs are formed

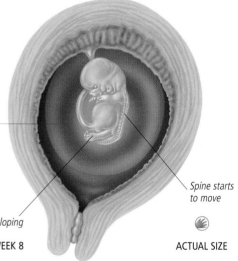

Spine starts to move

Limbs developing

WEEK 8

ACTUAL SIZE

THE DEVELOPMENT OF THE EMBRYO

Between weeks five and seven, the embryo develops physically at a rapid rate, though still very small. By week seven the intestines are formed and the limb buds are visible. The embryo is starting to look recognizably human. The small silhouettes represent the approximate size of the embryos.

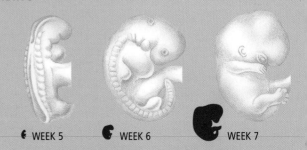

WEEK 5   WEEK 6   WEEK 7

but they are still solid. The inner parts of the ears and the eyes are developing. There are holes for the nostrils. Bone cells appear in what has thus far been cartilage bone. This marks the change from embryo to fetus.

Length: 15mm (¾in)

Week 8

All the internal organs are in place. The major joints of the shoulders, elbows, hips and knees are obvious. The spine can move. The genital organs are visible.

Length: 25mm (1in)

Week 9

The mouth begins to develop and the nose is formed. The limbs, hands and feet grow rapidly. Hearing has developed. Although you are unable to feel it, your baby is moving around quite a lot.

Length: 3cm (1¹⁄₁₆in)
Weight: 2g (¹⁄₁₆oz)

Week 10

The external parts of the ears are beginning to grow and the eyes are well formed. The head is still large compared to the rest of the body and its development is pronounced. The fingers and toes are distinguishable, but joined by webs of skin.

Length: 4.5cm (1¾in)
Weight: 5g (⅛oz)

Week 11

The ovaries and testicles are formed, as are the external genital organs. The heart pumps blood to all parts of the body. By the end of week 11 all the internal organs are fully formed and functioning. Only in rare cases now will these organs be harmed by infections, chemicals or drugs.

Length: 5.5cm (2³⁄₁₆in)
Weight: 10g (⁵⁄₁₆oz)

Week 12

Closed eyelids are distinguishable as the face becomes properly formed. Muscles are starting to grow on the body, which makes the limb movements more pronounced. Brain and muscles co-ordinate. Joints contract, toes will curl and the baby can suck. The fingers and toes are fully formed and have nails. The baby can swallow and takes in the amniotic fluid.

Length: 7.5cm (3in)
Weight: 18g (⅝oz)

Fingers and toes now have nails

Muscles are developing

WEEK 12

ACTUAL SIZE

Second trimester

The middle third of pregnancy is the time when you will feel the first fetal movements – about week 20 in a first pregnancy. Your baby is starting to look like a real person, with hair, even eyelashes, and to behave like one when he starts to suck his thumb. After week 24 of pregnancy the baby is considered legally viable, that is, capable of sustaining independent life with special care.

Week 13

Your baby is completely formed. During the rest of the pregnancy he mainly grows in size, so that by the time he is born his vital organs have matured to make him capable of independent life.
Length: 8.5cm (3½in)
Weight: 28g (1oz)

Week 14

The increase in weight is pronounced. Major muscles respond to brain stimulation. The arms can bend from the wrist and elbow; the fingers can curl and make fists. The heart can be heard with a sonicaid.
Length: 10.5cm (4in)
Weight: 65g (2¼oz)

Week 16

Limbs and joints are fully formed. Movement is vigorous, though rarely felt yet. Fine hair (lanugo) grows all over the body; eyebrows and eyelashes start to grow.
Length: 16cm (6in)
Weight: 135g (4¾oz)

Week 20

Your baby is growing very fast. The teeth are forming in the jawbone and hair is growing on the head. The muscles are increasing in strength. Movements are more vigorous and you should feel them by now. They are light flutters rather like bubbles bursting against your abdomen.
Length: 25cm (10in)
Weight: 340g (12oz)

Movements may now be felt

Ears and eyes are well developed

WEEK 20

ACTUAL SIZE

Week 24

The baby intermittently sucks his thumb and can cough and hiccup. He hasn't yet laid down fat stores and he's still thin.

Length:
33cm (13in)

Weight:
570g (1¼lb)

Head and body more in proportion

Baby can now suck thumb

WEEK 24

ACTUAL SIZE

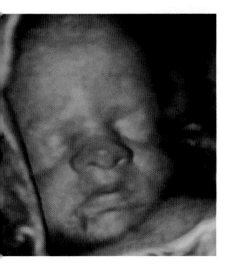

Week 28

The head is now more in proportion to the body. Fat stores are beginning to accumulate. The body is covered in thick grease (vernix), which prevents the skin becoming soggy from immersion in the amniotic fluid. The lungs are reaching maturity and the baby has a good chance of survival – about 80 per cent – if born.

Length: 37cm (14½in)
Weight: 900g (2lb)

Developing features
At this stage, the features are already becoming very like those of a newborn baby, as this coloured 3-D ultrasound scan of the face of a fetus at 28 weeks shows.

Third trimester

Your baby's organs are almost mature, except for her lungs. These aren't yet completely developed. If born during the third trimester before the 38th week, the baby might have breathing problems and difficulty keeping herself warm. However, with modern special-care facilities a baby has a good chance of survival – about 80 per cent at 28 weeks – and almost all babies born after 34 weeks survive.

Developing skills
By this time the baby can focus, although she won't need to develop this skill until after the birth. She can close her eyelids and she can blink.

Week 32
Your baby's proportions are as you would expect them to be at birth. She's much stronger and in over 90 per cent of cases she lies with her head down towards your pelvis. Her movements are now very vigorous and clearly discernible.
Length: 40.5cm (16in)
Weight: 1.6kg (3½lb)

Week 36
During the next four weeks the baby gains about 28g (1oz) a day. She fills the uterus and the movements are no less frequent, but are more like jabs as her space is

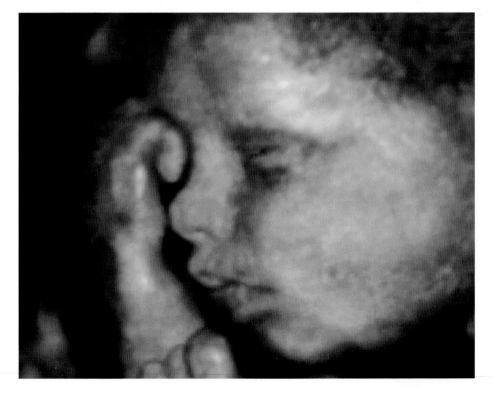

restricted and she settles into the position for birth. The irises of the eyes are blue or dark grey. The soft nails have grown to the end of the toes and fingers. Hair on the head can be up to 2.5–5cm (1–2in) long. In a boy the testes should have descended. The baby's swallowing mechanism should be established by now. If this is a first baby the head will usually descend into the pelvis around this time. With second and subsequent babies the head may not engage until later, or even until labour.

Length: 46cm (18in)
Weight: 2.5kg (5½lb)

Baby should now be lying head down

Movement now clearly discernible

Lungs are now mature

Head hair developed and could be 2.5cm (1in) long

WEEK 36

ACTUAL SIZE

Full term

Forty weeks after the first day of your last menstrual period your baby is ready to be born, though babies rarely arrive on the estimated day of delivery (*see p.27*). In these last weeks, your baby produces increasing amounts of a hormone called cortisone from his adrenal glands. This helps his lungs to mature and prepare him for his first breath.

Baby still moves but is too cramped to move freely

Head may now be engaged in your pelvis

WEEK 40

Week 40

The vernix has decreased so that there are only remnants in the skin folds – around the neck, armpits and groin. The nails on the fingers are long and will need cutting shortly after birth. When the baby is awake his eyes are open and he can discern light. Most of the lanugo has gone.

Length: 51cm (20in)
Weight: 3.4kg (7½lb)

ACTUAL SIZE

A tight fit
In this 3-D ultrasound scan of a full-term fetus, the head and a foot and hand are clearly visible. At this stage the baby has to lie curled up.

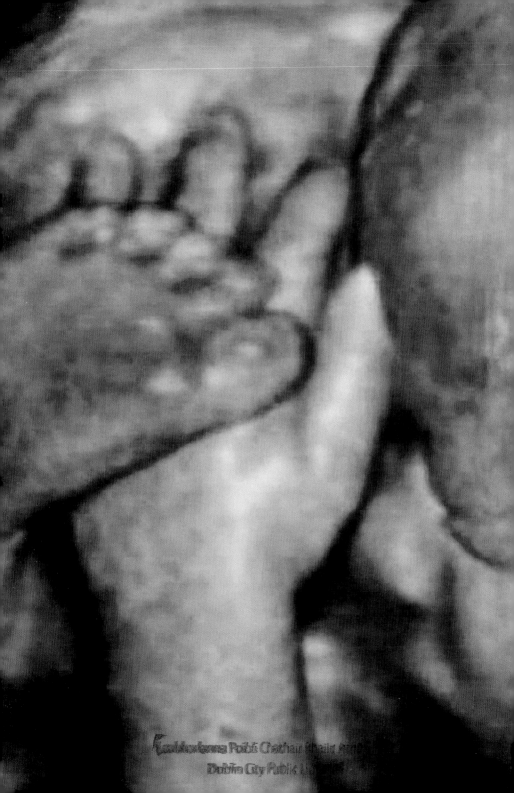

7 Physical changes

Nearly all the changes in your body that you can see and feel, such as bigger breasts, deepening pigmentation of the skin, and slight breathlessness on exertion, are due in one way or another to the increased production of pregnancy hormones. Early in pregnancy your ovaries are responsible for the main output, but very quickly the maternal supply begins to be overtaken by that from the placenta. The output of hormones is colossal – the output of oestrogen, for example, increases 20–30 times. These hormones cause changes in your whole body's structure and processes so that it can support and nourish your developing baby.

The menstrual cycle

The menstrual cycle begins when a hormone (follicle-stimulating hormone – FSH) from the pituitary gland stimulates the development of an egg (ovum) in a follicle inside one of the ovaries (see p.20). In a 28-day menstrual cycle (see p.18), ovulation happens around day 14 when the follicle bursts, discharging the ovum, which starts to move down the Fallopian tube towards the uterus. It is helped by "fingers" at the end of the Fallopian tube that direct it on its way and by fine hairs (cilia) within the tube.

At the same time, the lining of the uterus (endometrium) begins to thicken and the mucus at the neck of the uterus (cervix) becomes thinner so that the sperm can gain an easier entry. If the ovum is not fertilized, at around day 24 the decaying follicle (corpus luteum) begins to wither, and further hormonal changes result in shedding of the endometrium and bleeding on day 28 and day one of the next cycle.

If you do become pregnant, the ovum is fertilized around day 14 of the cycle, then implantation of the fertilized ovum in the uterine wall begins some seven days after that, around day 21. There are three or four days between implantation and the usual regression of the corpus luteum.

The body has only this short interval in which to stop the regression and suppress the menstrual cycle. This is probably achieved by a powerful hormone called human chorionic gonadotrophin (hCG), which is produced by the fertilized ovum and whose immediate function is thought to be the maintenance of a healthy corpus luteum and the levels of oestrogen and progesterone coming from the ovaries.

In this way, the mother's body and the developing embryo, which at this stage is only a minute ball of cells (*see p.20*), co-operate to keep the pregnancy intact.

The hormone levels of some pregnant women are not sufficiently increased to prevent some bleeding at the time of their first missed period. Slight breakthrough bleeding may sometimes happen at the time when the second and even third missed periods would have been due. The bleeding does not harm the baby. However, if the hormonal levels are too low, a miscarriage will almost certainly occur (*see p.158*).

The placenta

At implantation, part of the fertilized ovum puts out microscopic protrusions (chorionic villi) that embed themselves in the uterine wall. These villi become the placenta, which will supply food and oxygen to the baby and carry waste away.

During the first trimester, the placenta develops into an efficient chemical factory, producing an ever-increasing supply of hormones that alter the mother's body to maintain the pregnancy and prepare for lactation. They also maintain healthy reproductive organs and the efficient functioning of the placenta.

THE MONTHLY CYCLE

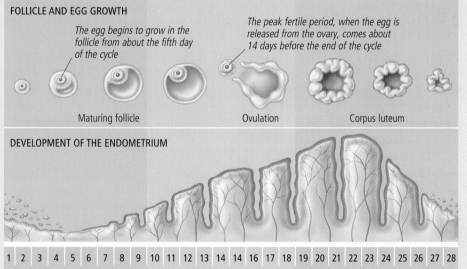

FOLLICLE AND EGG GROWTH

The egg begins to grow in the follicle from about the fifth day of the cycle

The peak fertile period, when the egg is released from the ovary, comes about 14 days before the end of the cycle

Maturing follicle   Ovulation   Corpus luteum

DEVELOPMENT OF THE ENDOMETRIUM

| 1 | 2 | 3 | 4 | 5 | 6 | 7 | 8 | 9 | 10 | 11 | 12 | 13 | 14 | 16 | 17 | 18 | 19 | 20 | 21 | 22 | 23 | 24 | 25 | 26 | 27 | 28 |

The cycle begins
The beginning of the ovarian cycle is signalled by menstruation, the shedding of the endometrium that lines the uterus. The hormone oestrogen controls the rebuilding of the endometrium.

Fertile period
After ovulation, under the influence of oestrogen and progesterone, the endometrium becomes thicker and spongy ready to receive a fertilized egg.

The cycle ends
If the egg isn't fertilized, the corpus luteum dies and, because oestrogen and progesterone levels fall, the endometrium is shed.

HORMONES OF PREGNANCY

Name	Action	Effect on mother and baby
Human chorionic gonadotrophin (hCG)	Produced by the chorionic villi. Causes the ovary to produce more progesterone, suppressing menstruation and sustaining the pregnancy. Maintains function of ovaries until placenta takes over.	High levels in the bloodstream parallel the time when women normally suffer from nausea in pregnancy (see p.25). Could be associated with morning sickness. Detection of this hormone in urine is a reliable pregnancy test (see p.26).
Human placental lactogen (hPL)	Produced by the placenta, it is essential to normal milk production.	Enlarges the breasts and causes secretion of colostrum from about the fifth month.
Relaxin	Probably produced by the placenta. In animal experiments, it was found to soften the uterine cervix.	May have an effect of relaxing the ligaments and joints, including pelvic joints.
Oestrogen	Produced in the placenta using starter substances from the mother's and the baby's adrenal glands.	Affects all aspects of pregnancy. It is particularly important in maintaining the health of the genital tract, the reproductive organs and the breasts.
Progesterone	Produced in the same way as oestrogen. Sustains the pregnancy, relaxes smooth muscle.	Affects all aspects of pregnancy. Prepares the breasts for lactation. Relaxes joints and ligaments and can affect bowel movements. Raises body temperature.
Melanocyte stimulating hormone (MSH)	Produced in higher levels than normal during pregnancy. Stimulates the skin to produce pigment.	Increase in colour of the nipples, patches of brown pigmentation on the face, inner thighs and a brown line running down the centre of the abdomen (see p.97).

Breasts

Changes in the breasts may be one of the earliest signs of pregnancy. Most women with an average 28-day cycle will notice a definite enlargement of the breasts by weeks six to eight of pregnancy (two to four weeks after their first missed period would have started). The breasts will feel firm and generally tender and have more and larger veins than usual running close to the surface of the skin. Tingling is common, as are occasional stabbing pains. The sebaceous glands on the areolas (Montgomery's tubercles) become raised, nodular and pink.

The breasts are composed mainly of millions of tiny milk glands, plus their small

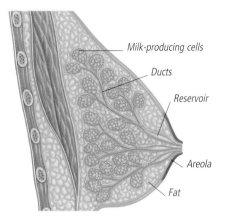

Milk-producing cells

Ducts

Reservoir

Areola

Fat

Cross-section of the breast
The breast is prepared for lactation during pregnancy. The milk-producing cells and ducts swell as a result of the oestrogen and progesterone in the body.

ducts, that join to come out at the nipple. Although there is almost certainly some overlap in the effect of hormones, oestrogen stimulates the growth of the ducts while progesterone stimulates enlargement of the glands themselves. From mid pregnancy your breasts will be making a form of milk called colostrum (*see p.221*). If you find yourself leaking colostrum try wearing breast pads.

Most of the growth of the ducts and increase in size and weight of the breasts happens in the first trimester. It is at this point that you should be fitted for a good bra. You will probably need one at least two sizes larger. After the baby is born, you'll also need feeding bras (*see p.135*). These should be fitted around a month before the baby is due. If you support the weight of your breasts during pregnancy and lactation they should return to their pre-pregnant shape and firmness when you stop breast-feeding. Some women find

their breasts are smaller after weaning as the original fat in the breasts has been replaced by milk-producing ducts. Towards the end of the first trimester you will see one of the last changes in the breasts, the darkening of the nipples and areolas due to a general increase in pigmentation (*see p.98*) – another characteristic of pregnancy.

Inverted nipples

If your nipples do not protrude when you're cold, sexually excited or breast-feeding, they are said to be flat or inverted.

You can improve inverted nipples by wearing breast shields under your bra from about week 15. Wear them for short periods at first, building up to several hours each day in the last trimester. An exercise known as the Hoffmann technique may also help. Place an index finger either side of the areola and stretch the nipples. Repeat this with your fingers placed above and below the areola. Do this a couple of times a day during pregnancy. Once you start breast-feeding, your baby may help to solve the problem but she could have difficulty latching on.

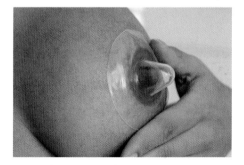

Flat or inverted nipples
Wearing special plastic nipple shields, also called breast shells, during pregnancy can help loosen the adhesions under the skin that stop the nipple protruding.

The uterus

Three principal tasks are performed by the uterus during pregnancy. It is the site of implantation by the fertilized ovum, it accommodates the growing baby, and it expels the baby at term. To achieve the second of these tasks the uterus has to grow and distend, while restraining a normal tendency to contract when there is something inside it and while the outlet, the cervix, remains resistant to stretching.

Expansion

To accommodate the developing baby, placenta and surrounding fluids, the internal capacity of the uterus has to expand from being about 5ml (¼fl oz) to around 5 litres (9 pints).

In the first half of pregnancy, the uterus gains weight quickly, mainly due to an increase in the size of the muscle fibres.

Each muscle cell of the uterus increases in size by as much as 50 times, initially under the stimulation of oestrogen. It'll start to press upon your bladder as it gets bigger, so you'll almost certainly need to urinate more often. But you probably won't notice your waistline changing until the end of the first trimester.

Around mid-pregnancy this rate of growth slows down, but uterine volume then increases rapidly. The uterus increases its weight some 20 times, from about 40g (1½oz) to 800g (2lb) at term. The expansion is not noticeable until about week 16 when the uterus begins to rise out of the pelvis. By week 36 of pregnancy the top of the uterus will have risen to just below the breast bone. When the baby's head engages in the pelvis (see p.169), it descends again.

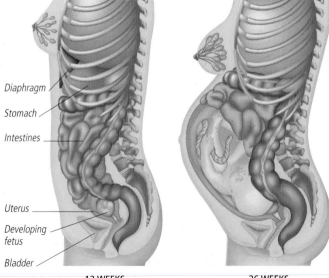

The expanding uterus
The uterus increases its capacity about 1,000 times in pregnancy and as it does so it puts pressure on other organs. This can cause problems such as frequent urination, heartburn, breathlessness and constipation.

Diaphragm

Stomach

Intestines

Uterus

Developing fetus

Bladder

12 WEEKS   **36 WEEKS**

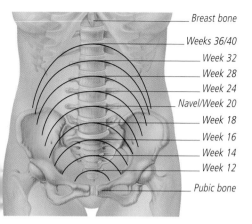

Breast bone

Weeks 36/40

Week 32

Week 28

Week 24

Navel/Week 20

Week 18

Week 16

Week 14

Week 12

Pubic bone

The height of the fundus
This can be determined by feeling the abdomen (abdominal palpitation) or by measuring in centimetres from the pubic bone. It is sometimes used as a guide to the duration of your pregnancy and the measurement may be written on your notes.

Contractions

One of the normal characteristics of uterine muscle is that it undergoes contractions that are hardly ever felt. All the way through pregnancy the uterus contracts in a weak, short-lived way that you may or may not notice, although if you put a hand on your abdomen you can feel the muscle going tight and hard.

These slight, painless movements are called Braxton Hicks contractions and occur about every 20 minutes throughout pregnancy. They are important as they ensure a good blood circulation through the uterus and help uterine growth. You probably won't notice Braxton Hicks contractions until the last month when they can be mistaken for labour.

Up until weeks 12–14, the developing baby can quite easily be accommodated in the space within the growing uterus, but after this time the junction of the uterus and the top of the cervix begins to smooth out, giving the baby more space. This part is called the lower segment of the uterus. While the upper half of the cervix is muscular and stretchy, the lower half contains a strong, tight band of fibrous tissue. This helps to prevent the cervix dilating before the baby is ready to be born.

Although this band of fibrous tissue softens during the last weeks of pregnancy to prepare for the birth, its resistance to dilatation is usually sufficient to withstand Braxton Hicks contractions. During labour, it is the upper segment of the uterus that contracts to push the baby out.

Vagina

Early in pregnancy, the vaginal tissues also change so that the vagina will dilate more easily for the birth. The muscle cells enlarge and the mucous membranes of the lining thicken. One side effect of this is an increase in vaginal secretions (*see p.152*), which may mean you need light sanitary pads for comfort. If the secretion has an

offensive smell or makes you sore, tell your doctor. Never douche during pregnancy. One other result of this increased lubrication and swelling of the vagina may be an increase in sexual pleasure. This, however, differs from woman to woman and will vary throughout the pregnancy (*see p.105*).

Vital functions

Your body will react to the hormonal stimulation of pregnancy with widespread changes in the important circulatory, respiratory and urinary systems. It used to be thought that the relationship between the mother and embryo was simply that of host and parasite, but we now know that it is much more complex than that. From the earliest days, in response to the diversified and raised hormonal output, the mother continually anticipates the needs of her baby: by changes in her vital functions, she precedes the baby's demands.

Blood

An average-sized, non-pregnant woman has about 5 litres (9 pints) of circulating blood. During pregnancy, the volume of blood increases by about 1.5 litres (2½ pints). The volume gradually increases from about week ten, reaching a plateau in the third trimester. The extra blood is required by the uterus (which takes about 25 per cent), the breasts and other vital organs – even the gums receive an increase in their blood supply *(see p.146)*.

The increase in the liquid part of the blood (plasma) is proportionately greater than that of the red cells. If the red cells become too diluted, this will show up in antenatal blood tests as a fall in the haemoglobin concentration – this is known as physiological anaemia. It is not the same thing as iron-deficiency anaemia *(see p.154)*. In a normal pregnant woman, the number of red blood cells multiplies steadily, particularly if you include a lot of iron in your diet.

Another effect of the increase of fluids circulating in the body is a lowering of the sodium concentration, which is why you shouldn't restrict your salt intake during pregnancy *(see p.111)* unless you have serious fluid retention.

Heart

With more fluids to push around the body, the heart has extra work to do when you're pregnant. By the end of the second trimester it has increased its workload by 40 per cent. It enlarges to accommodate this extra work, but astonishingly, your pulse rate is hardly raised from its pre-pregnant level. Much of the circulation increase is directed to the uterus.

Blood flow to the kidneys also increases as does the blood flowing through your skin, so that it is warmer and sweats more. During the third trimester, the uterus may press on the large vein in the abdomen if you lie on your back. This causes blood pressure to fall and may make you feel dizzy and faint.

Lungs

To keep your increased blood volume well supplied with oxygen, the lungs have to work harder than usual, too. Take plenty of fresh air and exercise, so that the blood supply to the lungs will be improved.

During the third trimester, the uterus will begin to put pressure on your lungs. You may feel uncomfortable, and find yourself having to take deep breaths. It helps to sit in a semi propped-up position whenever you can, even in bed, and try not to overdo things. Relief will come when your baby engages in your pelvis and there is less pressure on your diaphragm.

Kidneys

Your kidneys have to filter and clean 50 per cent more blood than they did before. As renal function becomes more efficient, the body gets rid of waste products like urea and uric acid faster than before. But the kidneys don't distinguish between waste products and nutrients, so glucose is also quickly cleared from the blood, together with minerals and vitamins – for instance, water-soluble vitamin C, plus folic acid that is excreted at four or five times the usual rate. This is one of the reasons for making sure your vitamin and mineral intake is maintained during pregnancy, and why you may need to take folic acid supplements (*see pp.12 and 112*).

In addition to the greater amount of urine to be eliminated, you will find you need to pass urine more often than usual as the expanding uterus presses on the neighbouring bladder. Even though you may find this very annoying, don't restrict your fluid intake.

Joints

The ligaments surrounding, connecting and supporting the joints are softened and become more flexible, especially in the pelvis, because of pregnancy hormones. In labour the pelvic joints stretch to allow the baby a smooth passage.

Joints affected include the sacroiliac joint (at the junction of the sacral bones of the lower back and the pelvic bones), and the symphysis pubis (junction of the pubic bones at the front). Increased fluid retention during pregnancy may cause movement of the symphysis pubis which can be painful. See a physiotherapist if you're affected by this.

After about week 16, the weight of the baby pushing down in the pelvis can tip the pelvic brim forward. The changed angle strains the muscles and ligaments of the lower spine, and may cause backache. You can counter this with good posture and by pelvic tilt exercises (*see p.122*).

Your legs and feet may also ache. Good posture (*see p.118*), regular exercise, wearing shoes with some support and having massages *(see p.143)* can do a lot to relieve discomfort.

Skin

All the extra hormones encourage the skin to hold moisture, which plumps out the skin, making it more supple, less oily and less prone to spots. The extra blood circulating around your body also makes your skin glow, but there can be problems, too. Red patches may get bigger, acne may worsen, areas may become dry and scaly,

and you may notice deeper pigmentation across your face. These changes usually disappear shortly after the baby's birth.

Pigmentation

Some degree of darkening is a universal characteristic of pregnancy, although its depth varies according to skin colour.

Blondes, redheads and even brunettes who have pale skins may see little change, whereas olive-skinned women may find that their whole skin darkens and areas like the nipples, abdomen and genital region remain dark brown after delivery.

Pigmentation of the nipples and areolas and a dark line down the centre of the abdomen, called the linea nigra, usually make their appearance around week 14. The linea nigra can be up to 1cm (½in) wide and stretches from the pubic hair to the navel, or even up to the breast bone. The navel tends to darken, and by the third trimester it stretches, becoming completely flat by 40 weeks. It returns to normal after delivery. The linea nigra also begins to fade shortly after delivery, but may take several months to disappear completely, or it may remain as a shadow.

Any brown birthmarks, moles, freckles or recent scars, particularly on the abdomen, may darken during pregnancy. The effect becomes more obvious after exposure to sunlight, but will probably return to normal shortly after delivery. Blotchy and irregular brown patches (chloasma) sometimes appear and are made worse by sunlight (see p.136). They usually begin to fade shortly after delivery and may disappear in a few months.

Texture

It's impossible to anticipate whether your skin, particularly on your face, will become drier or oilier, improve or get worse during pregnancy. High levels of hormones have several effects on skin, as does the greater amount of blood circulating to it. Oiliness results from the action of progesterone, which encourages the secretion of sebum.

Spots can appear unexpectedly because of fluctuating hormone levels, not just on the face, but on the back too. Increased fluid retention can fill out lines or it can cause unwelcome puffiness (see p.136), depending on your face shape. However, these changes are all normal and will disappear after your baby is born.

Stretchmarks

These occur in the skin under several different conditions. The first is in adolescence when we grow quickly. The second is whenever we put on a large amount of weight in a short time, and the third is during pregnancy. The underlying cause is always the same – tearing of collagen bundles. Collagen is the "skeleton" of the skin; its network of elastic bundles allows the skin to stretch with movement or with a change in size or shape. The marks in pregnancy are due to the high level of sex hormones that are circulating in the blood. One of the effects of these hormones is to break down and remove protein from the skin, thereby disrupting the collagen bundles and making the skin thin and papery. The skin appears delicate and stretchy in certain areas – the stretchmarks.

The stretchmarks that occur when we put on a lot of weight result when the collagen bundles are stretched to the point of breaking by the fat, which is laid down underneath the skin.

During pregnancy, these marks appear on the breasts, the abdomen, and also on the thighs and buttocks. They will remain pinkish throughout pregnancy, but after delivery they shrink and become a silvery colour after nine months or so (see p.150).

Hair and nails

These are both made from the same substance – keratin – and you may or may not notice any changes to your hair (*see also p.136*) and fingernails.

Hair changes

Pregnancy can have an unpredictable and quite dramatic effect on hair. Some women's hair becomes luxuriant and shiny, others' lifeless or greasy. Even body hair may become more or less apparent.

Most women's hair becomes more oily, particularly towards the end of the pregnancy, due to the very high levels of progesterone in the blood, which stimulate the sebaceous glands on the scalp.

If you've always had normal hair, you may find any change difficult to live with because your hair won't be as predictable as it was before. Because of this unpredictability, pregnancy is not a good time to dye your hair or have a perm.

One reason hair may become progressively thicker and stronger is that hormonal changes cause more than 90 per cent of the hair on your head to be thrown simultaneously into a growing phase (normally only 90 per cent is growing and the remainder resting).

Soon after birth the hair that you would normally lose, but didn't because of your pregnancy, will be lost in large amounts, making way for the new. Hair loss can go on for anything up to 18 months, which can be alarming, but rest assured, your hair will eventually recover. Your facial and body hair goes into a growing phase, too, which may increase its quantity and strength.

Nail changes

Splitting and breaking of nails is another problem for some women in pregnancy. Use rubber gloves and hand lotion to protect your nails. They will return to normal after delivery, although those who have stronger, shinier nails in pregnancy may suffer brittleness after delivery.

Teeth and gums

It used to be said that a baby absorbed the calcium from its mother's teeth and so women were more susceptible to tooth decay during pregnancy than at other times. This is not so, as there's no way of extracting calcium from the teeth. However, the high levels of progesterone during pregnancy will make the margins of the gums around the teeth soft and spongy, predisposing them to infection (*see p.146*). Be extra careful about oral hygiene and avoid the sugary foods that lead to tooth decay. See your dentist as soon as you know you're pregnant and have regular check-ups. Tell your dentist that you're pregnant as check-ups are free during pregnancy and for the year after giving birth. You should avoid X-rays.

8 Emotional changes

Psychologically speaking, your main task during pregnancy is to incorporate your new baby into your future. Though these challenges are similar for men and women, you can be affected differently. Any emotional turmoil you feel is a positive force to guide you through your period of adjustment and it's helping you to be emotionally prepared for your new baby. Having second thoughts doesn't mean that you've made a mistake. It would be wrong to think that having a baby is all fun. The best thing is to be open about your feelings. If you talk to each other honestly, you will clarify your thinking and prepare the basis for a constant exchange during the pregnancy.

Self-image

The changing size and shape of your body may make you feel strange about yourself. You might also worry that you're putting on too much weight, and that you'll look fat and unattractive either during or after your pregnancy.

Try to be positive about your changing shape. Look for the beauty in the fullness of your breasts and the curve of your abdomen. For both men and women, a pregnant body is extremely sensuous and a pregnant woman is beautiful in her own way. Your image of yourself in this condition is important. Feeling proud of your increasing curves and your fertility should make you more positive about your condition and encourage you to take a general interest in looking good (see pp.132–137), eating well (see p.110) and keeping fit (see pp.118–131).

How hormones affect mood

Mood changes are largely a reflection of the tremendous change in hormonal secretions, so there's no need to feel guilty about them. The upheaval of pregnancy makes nearly all women feel emotionally fragile, prone to crying and feelings of panic. It's normal to go through all these things because you're less in control of your feelings than usual. Even in the most positive of pregnancies you may feel some confusion. Once you know it's normal to feel low, you'll feel better and your moods will pass more quickly. Try not to be too analytical; react to the next thing that comes along.

Your changing shape
You should feel confident and proud of your rounded body: think of it as a reaffirmation of life.

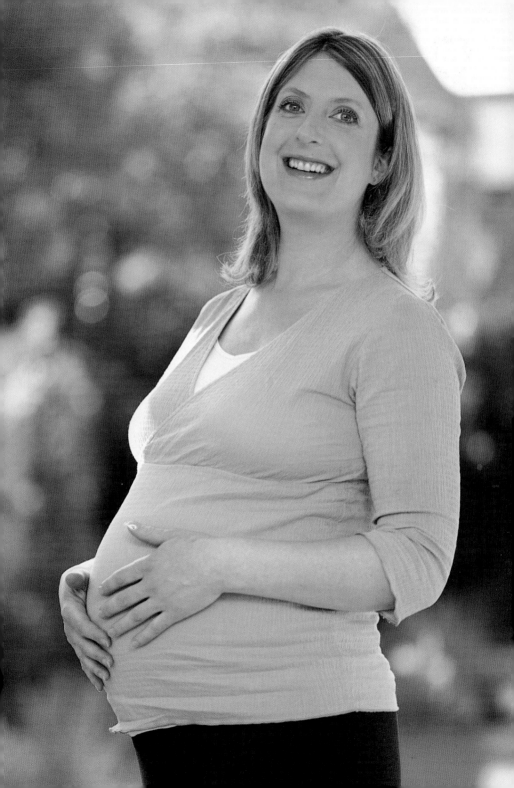

Feelings about your partner

The change from being an individual to being a parent is one of the most profound you'll ever experience; a woman is different from a mother; a father is not the same as a man. Approaching parenthood together is an essentially positive and deeply satisfying experience, but you're going to find it incredibly hard work too.

There are going to be many ups and downs for you and your partner to cope with during pregnancy. Be prepared for them and give them time and patience. If you're in a good partnership, one of the things that you'll almost certainly feel is that the pregnancy cements your relationship. If you can, try to go away for a weekend or have a holiday when you're between four and seven months pregnant (the time when most women feel at their best), as it will give you a chance to share your feelings and help you look forward to the exciting times ahead.

The strengthening of your bonds may be a little claustrophobic at first until you get used to it. It might help if you agree from the very beginning that you'll talk about things relating to the pregnancy in an open way and that you'll do your best to see things from each other's point of view.

During this time it's quite common for couples to make unusual demands on each other as a test of loyalty and devotion, but try to be realistic about small grievances and be quick to point them out and explain them to each other. The reality of approaching parenthood can sometimes cause tension, but this can usually be defused if you decide to be frank with each other. Friction and conflict seem to diminish when each partner is prepared to be generous towards the other.

You'll certainly start evaluating each other in the light of your new roles. You may have always had an image of the kind of parent you would want your partner to be and you'll try to see how he or she measures up to your fantasy. Don't be too hard on your partner; be sympathetic and think about how you would feel by evaluating yourself in the same way.

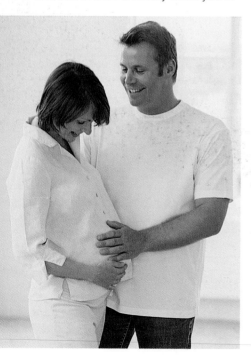

Increased intimacy
The special bond that pregnancy can bring often draws couples much closer together and helps them to strengthen their relationship.

BEING AN INVOLVED FATHER

Every father needs to take an active rather than a passive role in a fundamental life event such as the birth of his child. You need to feel that you really are contributing something as well and, even better, that you're taking this important step together.

Get involved from the beginning

Becoming a father doesn't start with the birth of your child: you need to get involved with the pregnancy from the beginning to understand what is going on in your partner's body and the physical and emotional pressures she is experiencing. Nearly all women are helped by the presence of their partner at the first antenatal visit, for example.

The golden rule is to be observant of your partner's needs, to assist in her care, and to be closely linked with everything that's happening to her. Fatherhood always involves hard work, a lot of responsibility and a considerable amount of time but will repay you with immeasurable joy, satisfaction and happiness. During pregnancy, the delivery and after the birth, your partner will be depending on you for courage and support. If she doesn't get them from you she will feel alone, which is bad for her and for your baby.

Some fathers-to-be feel jealous of their partner's growing bond with the baby. You may feel shut out if she seems more ready to talk about her pregnancy with her female friends. If you find that you are trying to minimize her needs, take a look at yourself. Make a special effort to be reasonable, and listen, sympathize and encourage. She'll almost certainly return your gifts, which means acceptance of you as lover and as the father of your child.

You need each other

The interdependence on one another is not easy in practice and certain traditions of male upbringing don't facilitate it. The strong, silent loner doesn't easily make an involved father. It's easier to learn from a good parent who acts as an example, but you may have to educate yourself into fatherhood.

It may hearten you to know that mothers and fathers start off more or less equally ignorant about babies, so don't be shy – get involved. Also, remember there's no one right or wrong way to be a parent, but you have to be ready to grow with your child – in caring, in admitting mistakes, and in making time for your family. All these things help to make you a better father.

Special anxieties

Nearly all prospective parents, but particularly mothers, are beset by anxieties about the baby, especially in the last trimester. The imminence of delivery and having a new baby nurtures natural anxieties about whether your baby will have any kind of abnormality, whether you will be a capable parent, whether you will do something silly like dropping your baby

and whether you will be able to cope with the day-to-day care. All of these feelings are quite natural and most women harbour them. If you know that they are going to occur but maintain perspective, this will help to defuse your anxiety.

Dreams in particular can be disturbing. You may dream of mistreating your baby or not caring for it properly. You may dream about losing the baby or that it is stillborn. Your dreams represent a perfectly legitimate fear that you have at the back of your mind, but which you are not prepared to face during your waking hours.

Dreaming can have a purpose

Think of your dreams as a release for your anxieties. Dreaming about harming your baby doesn't mean that you want to harm it or ever would; it's a healthy symptom of wanting to do the best for your baby.

Every pregnant woman at some stage worries about something being wrong with the baby. Dreaming about losing the baby or about having a stillbirth has little foundation in reality. It's more likely to do with figuratively losing the baby from your

uterus. Dreams about the baby dying are part of an understandable concern for the baby's well-being and are perfectly normal. They may be the brain's way of expressing feelings you may not be able to cope with or even be conscious about.

Concerns about labour

All women worry about how they'll behave in labour. Will the pain be too much? Will they scream? Will they lose control of their bowels or bladder? Such fears are normal and the chances are you'll be surprised at how calmly you'll behave, but most of us do something silly at some time during the labour and birth. Remember midwives and doctors have seen it before; nothing you do will shock or embarrass them.

Sex in pregnancy

The majority of women I've spoken to about sex and pregnancy have almost universally felt that sex was better than ever. Because of the high level of circulating hormones, a woman can become stimulated more readily and reach a high pitch of sexual excitement quicker than in the non-pregnant state. Many parts of her body, such as the breasts, nipples and genital area (see p.95), are more sensitive during pregnancy because all the sexual organs become highly developed and more capable of arousal than before pregnancy occurred. Also there's the freedom from having to think about contraception.

There does, however, tend to be some loss of libido during the first and third

trimesters. This could be a result of increased hormonal activity at the beginning of pregnancy, causing nausea and tiredness, and of your large shape at the end. Even if you don't feel like making love, and many couples don't, explore other ways of touching and giving sexual pleasure to each other.

There doesn't seem to be any medical reason why you shouldn't enjoy full sexual intercourse throughout your pregnancy, as the womb is completely sealed off by the mucous plug.

You can make love whenever you want to, provided you don't try to be too athletic and there aren't any medical reasons why you should avoid sex (see box right). Sex is good for your body too – orgasm exercises the uterine muscles, although this can cause contractions later on in pregnancy, which die down after a few minutes. Sex also helps you to become more aware of your pelvic floor muscles.

Lovemaking positions

You'll find that the missionary position becomes awkward and uncomfortable as your pregnancy goes on, but there are other sexual positions you can use. Side-by-side positions are often pleasurable, so is vaginal sex from behind, because in these your abdomen is not under any pressure from the weight of your partner. Sitting positions can be very enjoyable in the later months, allowing you to adjust your position but still see your partner's face and feel close to him.

Will sex harm the baby?

Your baby will be fine. Sex cannot introduce infection to the baby because it is safely protected in a surrounding bag of fluid. Sex will not crush the baby either. The bag of fluid (amniotic sac – see p.81) is an excellent cushion and once the baby is firmly attached to the mother's uterus, there's no way that intercourse can cause a miscarriage.

   If the baby should miscarry it will be for reasons other than the fact that you're having sexual intercourse. Likewise, your labour will not start simply because of the stimulation of sex.

Other ways of loving

If you're feeling sexy, but don't want intercourse, you and your partner could explore other forms of loving, such as erotically stroking and kissing one another, massage, mutual masturbation and oral sex.

WHEN NOT TO HAVE SEX

- If bleeding occurs, consult your doctor immediately and do not have sex. It may not be serious but your doctor has to rule out the possibility of placenta praevia (*see p.156*) or of miscarriage.
- If you have had a previous miscarriage, ask your doctor's advice or ask at your antenatal clinic. You may be advised to abstain during the early months while the pregnancy establishes itself.
- If you have a show (*see p.171*) or the waters break, there is a risk of infection.
- If you have placenta praevia.

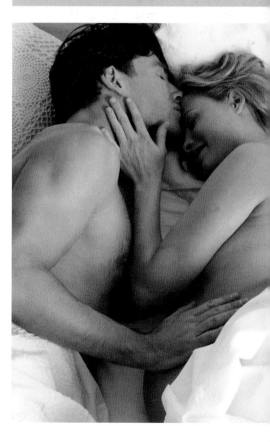

9 Health and nutrition

To ensure that your baby develops in a healthy environment, it's important to keep your body as fit and well nourished as you possibly can. It's not a question of devising a special diet for pregnancy, it's more to do with eating a good variety of the right foods – those that are rich in the essential nutrients. If you're deficient in any part of your diet, this can affect not only your health but also how well your body can support the pregnancy and nourish your baby. You also need to be aware of the risks posed by nicotine, alcohol and drugs as they can have a detrimental effect on the growth and well-being of your baby.

Weight gain

Nowadays it's known that you should gain a lot more weight in pregnancy than was thought healthy in the past. The amount of weight put on by women in pregnancy varies; on average women put on 9–14kg (20–30lb), with the most rapid gain usually between weeks 24 and 32. Your uterus, plus the baby, the placenta and the fluids will account for more than half of your total weight gain. You also manufacture more blood (see p.96) and you lay down fat to prepare for breast-feeding your baby.

I would not want to encourage anyone to gain an excessive amount of weight and you should forget the myth about "eating for two", but equally, dieting is not a good idea during pregnancy. It's much more important to eat a balanced and varied diet. A British study showed that there was a higher incidence of low-birthweight babies among those women who ate less than the recommended levels of calories, vitamins and minerals.

On the other hand, there's a lower incidence of physical and mental abnormalities, miscarriages and neonatal deaths when mothers have relatively high weight gain (although not when they become obese) and babies are born heavier. It has also been shown that prolonged labours are directly related to the way in which the uterus has grown during pregnancy, and that in turn is dependent on how well nourished the mother has been.

Eating well
A balanced diet that includes plenty of fresh fruit and vegetables will keep both you and your growing baby healthy during pregnancy.

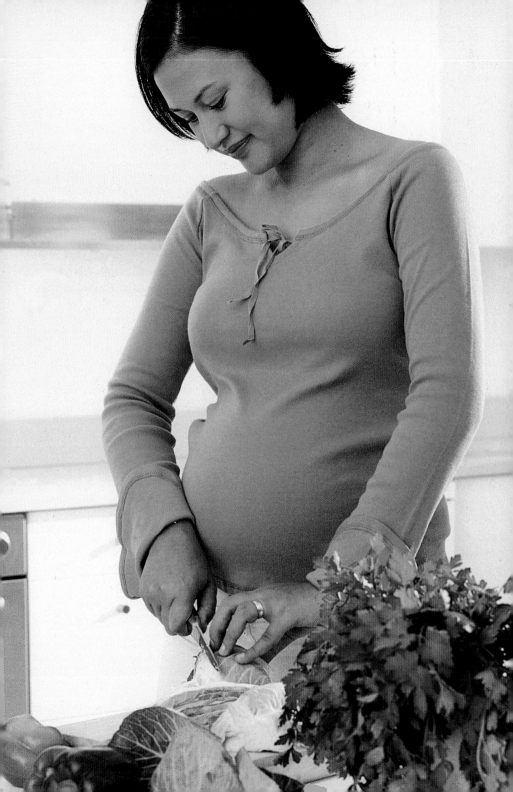

AWARENESS OF WEIGHT GAIN

If you're prone to plumpness during pregnancy, you may find you put on fat in places such as your thighs and upper arms. It's sometimes difficult to lose this fat again after the birth. As this is demoralizing, here are tips to help you keep your weight gain within reasonable limits.

• As soon as you know that you're pregnant, get someone to take a photo of you, and take one every month or so after that. This reminder of your changing shape will help you keep your size in perspective, and if you feel you might be putting on too much weight, this may help you to combat cravings for foods with a high fat or sugar content.

• If you've always had a tendency to weight problems, but managed to keep them under control, it's easy to relapse into over-eating once you know you're pregnant. Start eating sensibly from the beginning; try not to over-eat in the first trimester when your appetite will almost certainly increase, even if you suffer from nausea some of the time.

• Try to have regular, nutritious meals, and eat little and often later in your pregnancy. You're less likely to feel hungry in between.

• Keep a supply of nutritious snacks – cheese, fresh and dried fruit, wholemeal rolls – at home and at work. Avoid high-calorie, low-nutrition foods such as sweets, crisps and fizzy drinks.

• When preparing meals or snacks, follow these simple rules: eat unprocessed foods; include lots of roughage in your diet; grill rather than fry foods; sweeten with natural sweeteners.

• Don't eat to cheer yourself up. If thinking about your baby and the birth makes you too distracted to concentrate on any serious project that would normally occupy you, try going for a walk or do something such as a Sudoku puzzle to break up your routine.

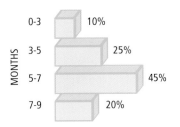

Percentage of total weight gain
This is a rough guide to your weight gain at a given time during pregnancy.

What you gain

Rather than emphasizing restriction, nowadays doctors consider that minimum weight gain for most women should be 11kg (24lb). When a woman eats what she needs, her weight gain usually follows a natural and predictable pattern. You may find you put on weight and your figure changes almost from the time you confirm the pregnancy (six to eight weeks).

Being overweight

Although there's no ideal weight gain to aim for, it's still not a good idea for weight gain to be excessive. True obesity presents problems: it puts extra strain on the heart, which is already working at full stretch, and there is an association between excessive weight gain and Caesarean section. There also appears to be links between obesity and complications in pregnancy. If you're definitely overweight and have been trying to lose weight, you should stop dieting when you decide to try for a baby. Unless your doctor considers you are dangerously obese, choose your foods with care when you're trying to conceive and once you are pregnant, but don't do anything drastic about losing weight until you've finished breast-feeding.

What to eat

Most of the daily food guides for pregnant women, with long lists of items to be prepared and measured out, don't take into account how busy most women are, or that they may not always be at home for meals. Rather than worry about exact portions, or lists, you should understand why you need certain foods and nutrients and work out your own plan for healthy eating. If you suffer from nausea, you may also have to plan when to prepare meals.

Your appetite will increase and by the fourth month of your pregnancy you may feel hungry all the time. This is nature's way of making sure that you take enough food for yourself and the baby. This doesn't mean you can "eat for two", however. Your energy requirements increase only by about 15 per cent, which means that 200–300 extra calories a day will be sufficient.

Every morsel of food you take in should be good for you and the baby. If you ate well before you became pregnant, you should be healthy enough to get through any period of nausea (*see p.148*). As your pregnancy progresses, try eating a greater number of smaller meals; small, frequent meals are always more easily digested.

Bowel contractions slow down during pregnancy so the stomach empties more slowly and should not be overloaded at any one time. Your developing baby pushes up into your stomach during the last trimester, constricting its capacity, so a small meal is more easily accommodated and you'll feel more comfortable. Keep healthy snacks, such as dried and fresh fruit, to hand.

FOODS TO AVOID IN PREGNANCY

As a general rule, foods have a higher nutritional value the less they are processed and cooked. Choose fresh, raw wholefoods wherever you can. When planning what to eat, remember:

- Processed foods with preservatives and colourings contain high levels of undesirable chemicals.
- White flour products or anything with added sugars provide little nutrition at the price of a lot of calories. Look at the list of ingredients on the labels of processed foods – you may be surprised how many savoury foods actually contain sugar!
- Sweet fizzy drinks – even the low-calorie versions – are not good for you. They provide few nutrients and may contain harmful additives.
- Strong coffee and tea adversely affect the digestive system. Caffeine in tea and coffee (also in colas and chocolate) is a stimulant and should be avoided. The tannin in tea interferes with iron absorption so drink organic herbal teas instead.

- Certain foods may harbour dangerous bacteria and should be avoided during pregnancy: pâté and soft cheeses (listeria), raw eggs (salmonella).
- Current advice is to avoid liver and liver products in pregnancy as the high levels of vitamin A they contain can be harmful for your baby.
- Avoid undercooked meat, unpasteurized goat's milk and goat's milk products. They may contain a parasite called toxoplasma, which can seriously harm an unborn baby.
- Avoid raw fish, especially shellfish, and don't eat shark, swordfish or marlin, which contain higher levels of mercury than other fish.
- Wash all fruits and vegetables thoroughly before eating or cooking to remove any traces of soil.
- Certain moulds produce toxic substances so don't eat mouldy foods. It's not enough to remove the mould as the harmful substances can penetrate deeper and aren't destroyed by cooking.

Vital nutrients needed in pregnancy

You shouldn't need to eat much more food than you did before you were pregnant, but you should be aware of the nutrients present in the foods you choose to eat.

Protein
Your protein requirements increase by 30 per cent during pregnancy. Your needs jump from 45–60g (1½–2¼oz) to 75–100g (3–4oz) of protein daily, depending on how active you are. Proteins are found in animal products – meat, dairy foods, fish, poultry and eggs – as well as in plant foods such as peas, beans and lentils, brewer's yeast, seeds and nuts.

Calories
During pregnancy you will need about 200–300 more calories a day than your usual requirement. You will get sufficient calories if you eat a varied, balanced diet.

You shouldn't have to concentrate deliberately on calorie counting – most women are too busy to do this anyway.

Fibre and fluids
As pregnancy progresses there is a tendency to develop constipation (see p.146). You can help to overcome it by giving your intestines plenty of roughage to work on. Raw fruit and vegetables, bran, wholegrains, peas and beans are all fibrous foods that you should eat some of every day.

When you're pregnant you have nearly 50 per cent more blood in your body than usual, so you need to keep up your fluid intake. Water is best, though fruit juice is also good. Drinking plenty also helps to avoid the risk of urinary tract infections. Don't cut down on your fluid intake if your hands and feet swell – it won't make any difference to this type of fluid retention.

VEGETARIAN DIET

Achieving a balanced diet with sufficient quantities of protein and all the vitamins and minerals doesn't require any more effort if you are a vegetarian. There are plant sources of protein that are complementary, so if you eat foods in combination you will gain all the necessary amino acids (the building blocks the body uses to make protein). For example, if you are eating grains – rice or corn – combine them with dried beans or peas or nuts. If your meal is made up of fresh vegetables, add a few sesame seeds, nuts or mushrooms to supply the missing amino acids. Few people eat one food in isolation anyway. There is relatively little iron in each helping of plant food, even leafy green vegetables and beans, and these foods often contain substances that interfere with the body's absorption of iron, so vegetarians need to make sure that they eat plenty of foods that contain iron.

Vegan diets
Pregnant women who don't eat any dairy products (vegans) need to ensure that their diet is rich in foods that contain calcium, vitamin D (or get plenty of sunshine) and riboflavin. The most difficult problem is adequate intake of vitamin B12, which is only found in animal sources. Very little is needed but lack of it will lead to a form of anaemia. Ask your doctor about taking synthetic B12.

Vitamins

Vegetables and fruits are good sources of many vitamins and minerals. Some are rich in vitamin C; others contain vitamins A, B, E, minerals and folic acid – all of which you need in your diet. Vitamins are quickly destroyed by exposure to light, air and heat and many can't be stored by the body, so you need to top up your supplies every day. Leafy green vegetables, yellow/red vegetables and fruit supply vitamins A, E, B6, iron, zinc and magnesium. Choose broccoli, spinach, watercress, carrots, tomatoes, bananas, apricots and cherries.

Some vegetables, such as watercress, are rich in many vitamins so are an excellent choice. Others provide a selection of vitamins and minerals, as well as fibre. It's particularly important to keep your levels of iron and calcium high to support your baby's development.

Although we can get some B vitamins from vegetables and fruit, the bulk of our intake comes from meat, fish, dairy products, grains and nuts. Some of the B vitamins are only in animal foods so vegetarians must make sure they're getting enough. If you don't eat dairy foods you may need vitamin B12 supplements, but check with your doctor. Vitamins can be toxic in large quantities so never take supplements without your doctor's advice.

Folic acid

This is essential for making red blood cells and plays an important part in the growth of your baby, especially during the first 12 weeks. Folic acid is essential to the development of the nervous system and research shows that folic acid supplements taken up to three months before conception and for the first 12 weeks of pregnancy significantly reduce the incidence of neural tube defects such as spina bifida. If you weren't taking folic acid before conception, start when you know you're pregnant. It is available in tablet form, and it's in cereals, bread and green leafy vegetables in the form of folate.

Minerals

A varied, healthy diet should provide you with enough minerals and trace elements – essential chemicals that help the body function properly but cannot be made by it. High levels of iron and calcium, in particular, are essential for your baby's development. Maintain a sensible salt intake in pregnancy – any excess is diluted by the increase in body fluids.

ARE YOU NUTRITIONALLY AT RISK?

If any of the following apply to you, you'll need to make a special effort to eat well during pregnancy and will almost certainly need supplements to maintain your health and the general health of your baby.
- You are allergic to certain key foods, such as cow's milk or wheat.
- Before conception you were generally rundown, underweight or eating a poor and unbalanced diet.
- You have had a recent miscarriage or stillbirth, or your children are spaced closely together.
- You drink or smoke heavily.
- You have a chronic condition that obliges you to take some form of medication constantly.
- You are adolescent and still growing.
- You have a multiple pregnancy.
- You have to work particularly hard or are subject to a lot of stress.

Iron and zinc

The body needs iron to make haemoglobin (the oxygen-carrying part of the red blood cells). When you are pregnant your iron intake must not only be adequate (*see opposite*) but also continuous. You need to keep up supplies of extra iron to support the large increase in the amount of blood in your body during pregnancy because your baby's need for iron is constant. Your body needs vitamin C to absorb iron.

Iron can block the body's absorption of zinc, which is essential for the development of your baby's brain and nervous system so

VITAMINS AND MINERALS NEEDED IN PREGNANCY

Name	Food source	What it does
Vitamin A (retinol)	whole milk, butter, cheese, egg yolk, oily fish, green and yellow fruit and vegetables	Builds up resistance to infection, essential for good vision, necessary for the formation of teeth, hair and nails, important for the growth and formation of the thyroid gland.
Vitamin B1 (thiamine)	whole grains, nuts, pulses, brewer's yeast, wheatgerm – benefits lost by overcooking	Aids digestion, keeps the stomach and intestine healthy, needed for fertility, growth and lactation.
Vitamin B2 (riboflavin)	brewer's yeast, wheatgerm, whole grains, green vegetables, milk, eggs – goodness can be lost if foods are exposed to light	Helps break down all food, prevents eye and skin problems, essential at the time of conception and early in pregnancy for normal development of the embryo.
Niacin (B3)	brewer's yeast, whole grains, wheatgerm, green vegetables, oily fish, eggs, milk	Builds brain cells, prevents infections and bleeding of the gums.
Pantothenic acid (B5)	eggs, wheatbran, whole grains, cheese	Essential for all normal reproductive functions, maintains red blood cells.
Vitamin B6 (pyridoxine)	brewer's yeast, whole grains, wheatgerm, mushrooms, potatoes, bananas, molasses, dried vegetables	Helps the body to assimilate fats and fatty acids necessary for the production of antibodies that fight disease; deficiency causes disease of the nerves and anaemia.
Vitamin B12 (cyanocobalamin)	brewer's yeast, wheatgerm, whole grains, milk, soya beans, fish, yeast extract	Essential for the development of healthy red blood cells, necessary for the formation of the baby's central nervous system.
Folic acid (one of B complex)	raw leafy vegetables, walnuts	Essential for blood formation, helps to prevent neural tube defects, such as spina bifida; essential for the development of the central nervous system.

you need zinc-rich foods, such as fish and wheatgerm, as well as iron-rich food.

Calcium

A baby's bones begin to form between four and six weeks, so you'll need plenty of calcium before you conceive and while you're pregnant. Dairy products, leafy vegetables, broccoli and fish containing soft, edible bones (such as sardines) are rich in calcium. If you don't eat dairy products, you may need supplements. Vitamin D is needed for calcium absorption so try to eat eggs or cheese every day.

Name	Food source	What it does
Vitamin C (ascorbic acid)	citrus fruits, fresh fruit, potatoes, red, green and yellow vegetables – destroyed by overcooking	Helps resistance to infection, builds a strong placenta, helps the absorption of iron from the intestine, a useful detoxicant in the body, important for the repair of fractures and wound healing. Needs are variable; infection, fever and stress deplete the body's resources and needs increase.
Vitamin D (calciferol)	fortified milk, oily fish, butter, egg yolk – sunshine activates a pre-vitamin in the skin	Promotes the absorption of calcium from the intestine and helps the incorporation of calcium from the blood and tissues into bone cells.
Vitamin E	wheatgerm, most other foods	Necessary for the healthy maintenance of cell membranes, also helps protect certain fatty acids.
Vitamin K	green leafy vegetables – manufactured by the body from bacteria in the gut	Aids in the process by which blood coagulates.
Calcium	milk, hard cheese, whole small fish, walnuts, sunflower seeds, green vegetables	Essential for the formation of healthy bones and teeth, important in the early months when the baby's teeth are developing.
Iron	kidneys, shellfish, egg yolks, red meat, molasses, apricots, haricot beans, raisins, prunes	Essential for healthy formation of the red blood cells. Can boost iron absorption by drinking orange juice with meals.
Zinc	wheatbran, eggs, nuts, onions, shellfish, sunflower seeds, wheatgerm, whole wheat	Helps in formation of many enzymes (special proteins that oversee chemical reactions in our bodies) and of proteins, needed to ensure the release of vitamin A from liver stores into the bloodstream.

Handy foodstuffs

Potatoes are very nutritious, so do include them in your diet. A potato contains about 3g (1oz) of protein, together with calcium, iron, thiamin, riboflavin and niacin, plus seven times as much Vitamin C as an apple. Try to cook potatoes in the skins; peeling them first means you lose fibre, most of the protein, many vitamins and half the iron.

Another useful food is milk; it is easy to use, a cheap source of protein, and provides calcium together with vitamins A and D. Skimmed or semi-skimmed milk contains the same amount of calcium as full-fat milk but fewer calories. If you don't like drinking milk, use it on cereals, soups and sauces, or eat cheese (two small cubes of cheddar are equal to one small glass of milk) or yogurt. If you are allergic to milk, substitute other sources of the nutrients it provides, especially calcium *(see p.113)*.

You'll see from the foods mentioned in this chapter that a few sources will provide the goodness you need for your own and your baby's health. Your daily needs are met by eating some of the following foods each day: milk or yogurt, eggs, fish, lean meat, yeast products, hard cheeses, wholegrain foods (brown bread, pasta or rice), fresh fruit and vegetables, fruit juices, nuts, dried fruits. Dark chocolate is good for a treat and it's rich in iron.

DIET AND MORNING SICKNESS

Ironically women who suffer from nausea in the first three months of pregnancy can be hungry at the same time. Food provides relief from the nausea, although the nausea soon returns. To combat this, many women find that small, frequent snacks and an avoidance of the trigger foods (usually rich, creamy or spicy foods) and smells (cigarette smoke, frying food) can help during the difficult weeks. Though called morning sickness, nausea can occur at any time of the day or even throughout the day. Work out your "good" times and prepare your meals and snacks then.

Eating more starch does seem to alleviate the sick feeling. But instead of eating cakes and biscuits, have nutritious forms of carbohydrate such as wholemeal bread, rice and potatoes. Here are some snacks to keep at home and at work:
- slices of dried wholemeal bread
- wholemeal-bread cheese sandwiches

- nuts and raisins
- dried apricots
- fruitcake (preferably made with wholemeal flour and wheatgerm added)
- crisp green apples
- water crackers and cottage cheese
- raw vegetables such as carrots, celery, tender young green beans, peas from the pod, tomatoes
- diluted fresh fruit juices
- carbonated water with a slice of lemon
- bitter lemon or lime
- diabetic peppermints (suck them slowly)
- commercial muesli bars with bran, coconut or apple added
- unflavoured, natural yogurt with honey
- fruit sorbet
- herbal teas, especially mint tea
- soft, juicy fruits such as peaches, plums and pears
- milkshakes made with skimmed milk.

Dangerous substances

If you normally smoke or drink, change your habits – preferably before conception – to protect your unborn baby. You also need to take extra care with hygiene, particularly when handling raw meat and when cleaning out cat litter. Raw meat and cat faeces contain a parasite, toxoplasma, that can damage your unborn child.

Smoking

- The chemicals absorbed from cigarette smoke limit fetal growth by reducing the number of cells produced, both in the baby's body and brain. Nicotine causes blood vessels to constrict and so reduces the blood supply to the placenta, interfering with the baby's nourishment.
- The level of carbon monoxide is higher in a smoker's blood, and whatever the level in the woman's blood, it's higher in her baby's blood. As well as being a poison, carbon monoxide reduces the amount of oxygen that blood can carry. The more carbon monoxide in the baby's blood, the lower its weight at birth. The babies of mothers who smoke can be as much as 200g (7oz) lighter than those of mothers who don't smoke, and low birthweight babies can have problems and are less likely to survive. The incidence of prematurity almost doubles in smokers.
- Studies have shown that smokers are more likely to have children with all types of congenital malformations, especially cleft palate, hare lip and central nervous system abnormalities, with the risk more than doubled in heavy smokers.
- Smokers have nearly twice the risk of

miscarriage and stillbirth, partly because smoking greatly increases the risk of the placenta detaching itself from the wall of the uterus (see *p.156*), and partly because smokers' placentas tend to be thinner and age prematurely.

- Neonatal deaths are more common among babies whose mothers smoked. Mothers who continue to smoke after the fourth month are increasing the risk of their baby dying by nearly one third.
- The effects of smoking in pregnancy last for a long time after your baby is born, and children who live in smoking households are less healthy than others in many respects.

SMOKING AND PREGNANCY

Here are some of the facts about smoking and pregnancy.

- Stop smoking three months before trying to conceive – men and women.
- If you need to feel something in your mouth, chew sugar-free gum.
- If you smoke when you're pregnant you risk harming your unborn baby, having a miscarriage or giving birth to an underweight baby who is vulnerable to infections.
- The children of men who smoke 20 or more cigarettes a day have a higher risk of cancer than children of non-smokers. Smoking damages sperm, so prospective dads should give up.
- Smoking increases the likelihood of SIDS.
- No one should smoke in a house where there is a baby or young child and don't let anyone who is smoking hold your child.
- Passive smoking increases risk of miscarriage.

• Exposure to cigarette smoke puts babies at considerable risk during the first year of life – they have a tendency to develop bronchitis and the incidence of SIDS (cot death) increases.

Dangers of smoking

All smoking is dangerous for your unborn child. The only safe option is for both you and your partner to give up smoking at least three months before you conceive. Women who live with smokers or who are often in a smoky environment, are at risk even if they never smoke themselves. The children of fathers who smoke heavily are twice as likely to have malformations.

Drinking alcohol

The extent to which alcohol, a poison, can seriously damage a developing baby has only been appreciated in the last ten or so years. Some of the alcohol of every drink you take reaches your baby's bloodstream and is most harmful during the critical development period of weeks six to 12, although each affected growth period seems to produce its own abnormalities.

There is no safe level of alcohol consumption in pregnancy. If you have more than two drinks a day, there is a one in ten chance that your baby will have Fetal Alcohol Syndrome (FAS), which can lead to facial abnormalities, such as cleft palate and hare lip, heart defects and abnormal limb development, in addition to lower than average intelligence and behavioural problems.

Babies seriously affected by FAS never catch up mentally or physically with their counterparts. Binge-drinking can cause the same damage, even if you drink little as

a rule: one incident of excessive alcohol consumption is just as capable of giving rise to FAS as drinking excessively all through pregnancy.

It has been shown that as little as one unit of alcohol a day can double the risk of having a small-for-dates baby, and babies of women drinking half that amount tend to be shorter than expected. It is also thought that very small intakes of alcohol can cause many mental conditions so far unexplained, or affect babies mentally and physically in subtle ways. In the light of all this, it seems best for pregnant women to avoid alcohol altogether *(see p.13)*.

Drugs

It's well known that certain drugs can affect the development of a baby, particularly at the sensitive period between weeks six and 12 when all the vital organs are being formed. A drug may be safe in itself, but it can be harmful to the fetus if taken in combination with another equally innocent drug or certain foods.

Because of these dangers no drug of any kind, and that includes aspirin, should be taken unless under the supervision of a doctor. Don't take over-the-counter remedies for anything, or use leftover prescription drugs, or accept drugs prescribed for other people. And don't consult a doctor about anything without informing him or her that you are pregnant or trying to become pregnant.

Some drugs have to be taken for the treatment of chronic complaints *(see p.15)* such as diabetes, heart disease, thyroid problems, rheumatic disorders and possibly epilepsy. You should discuss any medication with your doctor before you conceive.

EFFECTS OF DRUGS ON YOUR BABY

Drug Name	Effects
Amphetamines	Stimulants. May cause heart defects and blood diseases.
Anabolic steroids	Body building. Can have a masculinizing effect on a female fetus.
Anti-inflammatories	Can cause premature closing of an important valve in baby's circulatory system.
Antibiotics	Most are safe but may cross the placenta. Only take on doctor's advice.
Tetracycline	Used for long-term treatment of acne. Avoid because it causes permanent yellow discoloration of the baby's teeth and may interfere with growth of bones and teeth.
Streptomycin	May cause deafness in infants. It is used to treat tuberculosis.
Antihistamines	Some may cause malformations so only use with medical supervision.
Anti-nausea drugs	May cause malformations (especially Thalidomide, although this is hardly ever prescribed these days: never, ever take while pregnant). Check with your doctor.
Aspirin	Can cause problems with blood clotting, but may be used for some causes of recurrent miscarriage.
Contraceptive pills oestrogen/ progesterone	Can cause malformations of the limbs, defects of the vital organs and masculinization of the female fetus. Best to stop taking the pill at least three months before conceiving (*see p.16*).
Codeine	Used in pain relief and in some cough medicines. Increased incidence of malformations, such as cleft palate and hare lip, has been reported. Codeine is an addictive drug, which can cause withdrawal symptoms in the baby at birth.
Diuretics	Used to rid body of excess fluid. Can cause fetal blood disorders.
Paracetamol	Reduces fever. Safe in small doses.
Progestogens	Taken by mouth accidentally may cause fetal masculinization. Generally now only used in assisted conception clinics.
Street drugs	Risk of chromosomal damage, and miscarriage.
Sulphonamides	Can cause jaundice at birth. Used to treat urinary infections.
Tranquillizers	Some of the stronger types may affect growth and development, causing malformations. Check with your doctor but best to avoid in pregnancy.

10 Exercise

Both before and during pregnancy, exercise is essential. Before pregnancy, it ensures that your body is fit to carry a healthy baby to term. Once pregnant, it strengthens muscles to protect your joints and spine, which slacken prior to labour and ache when over-used. Specific exercises, when combined with breathing and relaxation techniques, help conserve energy in labour, while others prepare you for delivery positions.

Being aware of your body

Your body changes in many ways during pregnancy. There are the obvious physical changes *(see pp.90–99)*, as well as the loosening up and stretching of the ligaments around the joints. But more important, on a day-to-day basis, is the difference in what your body can do with ease compared to what it could do before.

In later pregnancy you become a rather ungainly shape and many women find they lose some agility and mobility, becoming breathless more easily. Your centre of gravity is further forward and you're less stable. To compensate for this lack of stability, you might try holding your shoulders back, stand with your feet apart, and walk with a waddling gait.

These compensatory actions mean that you're using muscles in a different way and may therefore suffer minor aches and pains as pregnancy progresses. If, however, you keep your body fit during pregnancy, and protect it from stresses and strains, the muscles, joints and ligaments will take the

strain more easily, without aching. You may even avoid minor discomforts altogether. Get used to thinking that your body is in a special, not an abnormal, state, and develop reflexes and postures that take account of its needs. If you do feel

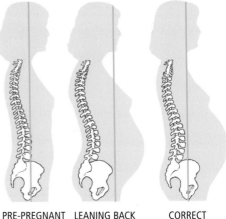

PRE-PREGNANT   LEANING BACK   CORRECT

Correcting bad posture
Your centre of gravity changes as the baby grows; women often lean back to compensate (centre). Good posture (right) corrects balance and lessens backache.

uncomfortable, ease your discomfort by practising some simple relaxation techniques *(see p.140).*

Bending and lifting

Pregnancy hormones soften the ligaments of the lower back and pelvis, so avoid heavy lifting in order to protect your spine and avoid unnecessary strain.

• Make use of your thigh muscles when lifting. Squat down first, keeping your back straight. Prepare your body (keep your feet slightly apart) by tensing your abdominal muscles, pulling up your pelvic floor muscles *(see p.122)*, taking a deep breath and counting to three before lifting on four. As you lift, breathe out. Stand close to whatever you're lifting and keep it close to your body as you pick it up.

• When you're carrying anything, avoid swivelling to either side. Try to distribute your weight evenly as, for instance, with heavy bags of shopping.

• When you're carrying your toddler keep your body straight, don't twist, and change him from side to side.

• If you have to do anything that involves being low down, squat *(see p.129)* or get down on all fours. This is a comfortable position, particularly if you suffer from backache, as it takes the weight of the uterus off your spine.

• If you have bad posture, or your back isn't flexible, improve your suppleness by sitting cross-legged against a wall. Lengthen your spine, and tilt your pelvis, pressing your back into the wall. This helps to strengthen your spine.

• Avoid lifting anything heavy down from a height. Your back will arch and you could lose your balance if the object is heavier than you thought.

PROTECTING YOUR SPINE

In later pregnancy you need to adapt all your movements, even basic everyday ones like getting up from lying down, getting out of a chair or lifting things. You want to put the least strain possible on your back and let your thighs do the work.

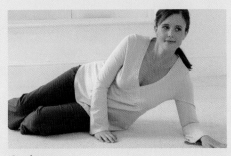

Getting up
Roll on to your side and use your arms to push yourself up sideways.

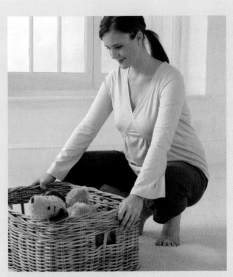

Picking up heavy objects
Remember to keep your back straight and to bend your knees.

Keeping active

Pregnancy, labour and delivery will make great demands on your body, so the more you can prepare yourself physically, the better. Whether you do this by continuing to exercise in the way you did before pregnancy or whether you start a new form of exercise is up to you. The most important thing is to keep yourself active. The fitter you are, the less likelihood there will be of your stiffening up as pregnancy progresses. If you sit, stand and walk in the correct ways *(see pp.118–119)*, you should avoid the aches and pains that invariably come with bad posture.

The benefits of being fit

Regular exercise will improve your mental as well as your physical well-being. Exercise causes the body to release endorphins, the body's natural painkillers, helping you to relax and soothing away tensions and anxiety. And the boost in blood circulation that occurs when you exercise means that your body and your baby will be well oxygenated. Labour will almost certainly be easier and more comfortable if you have good muscle tone, and many of the exercises taught in antenatal classes, combined with relaxation and breathing techniques, will help give you more control over what is happening to you.

Keeping in condition during pregnancy will also mean that you regain your normal shape more quickly after delivery, and regular exercise of the pelvic floor muscles *(see p.122)* will not only assist in delivery, but will also allow your muscles to regain their normal strength more quickly.

However, before you start on any exercise programme in early pregnancy, check with your doctor to make sure it is safe. When you have the "all-clear", here are a few tips for keeping fit:

- Try to enrol in an exercise class specially designed for pregnant women. Many women find it easier to exercise regularly this way as they have the motivation of a teacher putting them through the exercises. It also helps to have someone watching you, correcting the way in which the exercises are done.
- If you haven't been an active person before pregnancy you're unlikely to change dramatically during it, but at least try to walk whenever you can, 20 minutes a day if you can manage it.
- If you have to sit at work all day, there are exercises that you can do in a chair to help keep you supple *(see p.127)*.
- Get into the habit of going through a 10–15 minute exercise programme every day. During pregnancy, exercises should be regular and taken at a slow pace. They should be rhythmic whenever possible, so it helps to exercise to music.
- Always warm up gently before you start your exercise programme *(see p.124)*.
- Try not to go for periods of time with no exercise at all. A little exercise several times a day is better than a big burst followed by a long gap.
- Never do any exercise that hurts. Pain is a signal that something is wrong. Try a simpler variation of the exercise. Work towards a position gradually, and don't strain.

- Never exercise to the point of fatigue.
- Try not to point your toes for too long when you're working out as it may cause cramps in your legs.
- Most exercises are done on the floor so use a yoga mat and a few cushions to make yourself comfortable.
- Before each exercise, take a few deep breaths. This is relaxing, it makes you feel alert, it gets the blood flowing around your body and gives all your muscles a good supply of oxygen.

Antenatal exercise classes

A variety of antenatal exercise classes are available and it's worth doing some research into what they have to offer. The hospital or clinic will run classes (*see p.69*) or there are independent organizations and workshops specially for pregnant women.

What they teach
Some classes are run just like an ordinary exercise class, giving a thorough physical workout with exercises specifically designed for pregnant women to increase flexibility, strength and stamina. Others are designed with a certain philosophy of birth in mind. If you want to give birth in a squatting position, there will be exercises to strengthen your back and thighs, for example. The classes are also good places for meeting other pregnant women.

Yoga
With its emphasis on muscular control of the body, breathing, relaxation and tranquillity of mind, yoga is an excellent method to use as a preparation for pregnancy. However, yoga is a philosophy that pervades the whole of life and, although special exercises for pregnancy exist, they are only a small part of the system. If you are a devotee or have done some yoga-based exercises prior to your pregnancy, yoga can be of great help.

Yoga exercises are comparable to those taught in antenatal classes but the breathing used is different. It's thought that these breathing techniques help to raise the pain threshold.

Mind and body
Relaxation techniques and yoga exercises prepare you both mentally and physically for the birth by keeping you supple and fit and improving breathing techniques.

The pelvic floor muscles

The muscles that make up the pelvic floor support the uterus, bowel and bladder, rather like a sling holding the pelvic organs in place. They lie in two main groups, forming a figure of eight around the urethra, vagina and anus. The muscle fibres originate front and back from high up on the pubic and sacral bones. The layers of muscle overlap and are therefore thickest at the perineum.

The action of progesterone

The pregnancy hormone progesterone prepares the body for birth by softening joints and ligaments, and that includes the pelvic floor muscles. If pressure from the enlarging uterus causes the pelvic floor to become weak, this can lead to vague aches and fatigue, to urinary incontinence and leakage, and possibly, at worst, even to prolapse of the uterus after childbirth. About half the women who have had children later suffer from some weakness of the pelvic floor and may have "stress" incontinence – slight leakage of urine when they laugh, cough, sneeze, or lift.

To counter this, a set of exercises to strengthen the pelvic floor muscles has been developed by physiotherapists working in the area of childbirth. They are known as the Kegel exercises, after Dr Arnold Kegel of the University of California in Los Angeles, one of the first physicians to recognize how important these muscles are. Pelvic floor exercises are recommended for all women. It's best to begin doing the exercises before pregnancy and continue afterwards (they are probably even more important in older women). If you possibly can, make the exercises (*see opposite*) part of your daily routine.

When exercising, do about five contractions of five seconds each. Once you've mastered the exercises, you can do them wherever you are – sitting at home, standing in a queue or walking – but do

PREPARING FOR THE BIRTH OF THE BABY'S HEAD

Having an increased awareness of the pelvic floor muscles and how they feel when relaxed will help prepare you for the birth of your baby's head.

Exercise one
Lie on a bed, your back supported, but your feet and knees apart. Gradually relax your thighs and pelvic floor muscles so that your knees fall wider and wider apart (your feet will roll gently onto their outer edges). Practise panting in this position as the midwife will ask you to do when it's time for your baby's head to pass gently out of the birth canal.

Exercise two
Lie on a bed with your knees bent, feet together and your back supported. Press your knees together hard and tighten your pelvic floor muscles at the same time. Notice the feeling of tension along your inner thighs and between your legs; many women involuntarily tense these muscles when their baby's head is stretching the outlet of the birth canal.

Now relax your muscles, and this time notice carefully the different feel of your muscles. This open feeling is what you should aim for when you're giving birth.

remember to practise as often as you can. They will also be useful in the second stage of labour when the baby's head is about to be born *(see box opposite)*.

Locating the pelvic floor muscles

Lie down with a pillow under your head and one under your knees. Cross one leg over the other and squeeze your legs tightly together. Tighten the buttock muscles and pull up as if you feel the need to empty your bladder but must wait. This helps you find your pelvic floor muscles, which you'll feel tighten inside your vagina.

Another way to locate the muscles is to interrupt the flow mid-stream when you pass urine, because the muscles that control the flow of urine are your pelvic floor muscles. Only do this to find out where the muscles are and always empty your bladder completely afterwards. When doing the exercises *(see opposite)*, ignore the abdominal and buttock muscles and use only those of the pelvic floor.

Isolating the sphincter muscles

Lie down as above but with your legs relaxed and not crossed. Place a clean fingertip on the opening of your vagina and contract your pelvic floor muscles. You will be able to feel the contraction of the vaginal sphincter. The sphincter at the opening of the urethra is more difficult to isolate than the pelvic floor muscles because of its proximity to the vagina. But the sphincter muscles are also tightened when you contract the pelvic floor muscles. Now place your finger at the opening of your bowels and, with a larger movement, contract the muscle around the anus. You will feel the anal sphincter tightening.

PELVIC FLOOR EXERCISES

Here are three basic Kegel exercises that will help you to strengthen your pelvic floor muscles and keep them well toned during pregnancy.

Contract and release

Lie on your back with your legs apart. Draw up the pelvic floor muscles, concentrating hard on the muscles of the vaginal sphincter. Hold this position for two to three seconds and then completely relax. You can try to slacken the muscles a little more and notice the release in tension. Do three of these contractions in succession.

The lift

Imagine the pelvic floor is a lift, stopping at various levels in a department store. Aim to contract the muscles gradually in five stages with a short stop at each level, not letting go between levels. Then allow the pelvic floor to descend, releasing the contraction level by level. When you reach the starting point, ground level, allow the pelvic floor muscles to relax completely so that you feel a slight bulging downwards. If you actually push downwards below this level you can lower the pelvic floor even further, and the vaginal lips will open slightly. To do this you need to hold your breath or blow out and then you should be able to feel the lips of the vagina opening. This is the position in which your pelvic floor should be while your baby's head is being born.

During sex

Grip your partner's penis with your vagina. Hold for a few seconds before releasing. Repeat this exercise a couple of times. Your partner can tell you how hard you're squeezing and will know when the strength of the squeeze is diminishing. If he can't feel much, then you will know that you need to do the exercises more frequently.

Stretching

Always precede your exercise programme by warming up with these few stretching exercises. They gently warm up the muscles and joints so that you can move more freely, reducing the risk of overstretching and damage. Warming up muscles before exercising will also reduce the risk of you suffering from stiffness and cramp. Furthermore, these exercises help to stimulate the circulation, giving you and your baby a good supply of oxygen. Repeat each exercise five to ten times; work on a firm surface, make sure you are comfortable and that your posture is good with your back straight. If necessary, lean your back against a wall or use cushions for extra support. Remembering to breathe normally throughout, start the routine slowly and if you feel any pain, discomfort or fatigue, stop at once.

Place your left hand on your right knee to help control the stretch

Gently turn to look over your shoulder, keeping your back and neck straight

Breathe out as you turn to the left, stretching as far as is comfortable

Waist and thigh stretches
Sit with your back straight, bend your knees and bring the soles of your feet together; breathe in deeply. Then cross your legs, breathe out and turn your upper body towards the right, placing your right hand behind you and put your left hand on your right knee. Hold for a count of five. Then repeat to the other side.

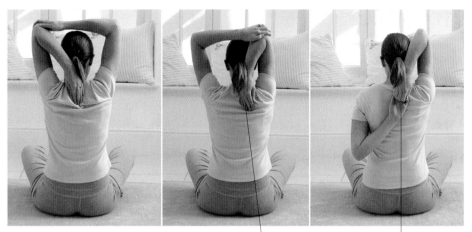

Arm stretches

Lift your left arm up above your head. Bend your elbow, and drop your hand down behind your back. Put your right hand on your left elbow and push it gently. Repeat with the other arm. Then, put your right hand down behind your back and reach up to grasp it with your other hand.

Reach as far down your back as you can. Don't strain

Clasp your hands together. Don't worry if you can't quite reach

Leg and foot stretches

Toning the calves and feet will help to prevent cramp, a common problem in pregnancy. Sit with your legs stretched out in front of you. Slowly raise one knee, hold for a count of five and then straighten out the leg. Repeat with your other leg. Then raise your foot off the floor and flex it outwards. Circle your ankle in both directions. Relax and repeat with the other foot.

Place your hands by your hips to support your weight

Flexing your foot towards your body helps to increase the stretch

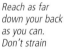

Floor exercises

Stretching different parts of the body relieves strain and tones vital muscles. Strengthening the lower back is particularly important, and helps to prevent backache. By working on a firm surface and carrying out all movements smoothly, you shouldn't feel discomfort or strain. These exercises can easily be fitted into your day. Repeat each one five times to begin with, increasing slowly until you're doing 10 or 15. Don't, however, do these exercises after week 32 of pregnancy. At this late stage it's not a good idea to lie flat on your back for any length of time as the pressure of the uterus on deep veins in your pelvis may result in fainting and dizziness.

Pelvic lift

Lie flat on the floor with your arms by your sides. Pressing your feet into the floor, squeeze your buttocks and lift your pelvis up into the air as high as you can. Hold for a count of five. Gradually lower your back down one vertebra at a time.

Lower your back gradually, let your thigh muscles do the work

Relax and don't hold your breath

Lower back release

Lie flat with your arms by your sides. Keeping your lower back in contact with the floor, bring your knees to your chest, and grasp them with your hands. Hold for a count of ten. Inhale, then breathe out as you raise your pelvis. Hug your right leg, straighten your left leg and lower it to the floor. Repeat with opposite legs.

Very gently pull your knees towards you

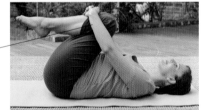

Hold for a few moments

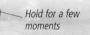

SITTING EXERCISES

It's easy to neglect parts of the body like the neck or the ankles. These exercises here will keep you supple and help prevent the build-up of fluid (oedema) that causes puffiness, especially in the ankles. You can do them anywhere: try them in the evening as you sit watching TV.

Head and neck

Sit cross-legged and tilt your head to one side. Lift your chin, rotate your head back, over to the other side and down in one flowing movement. Repeat in the opposite direction. Then, keeping your head straight, turn it to the right and to the left. Return to face the front.

Rotate your neck slowly and carefully to avoid injury

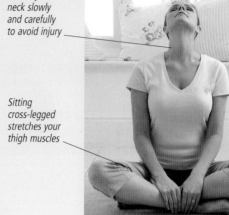

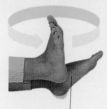

Circle five times to the right

Ankles

Sit barefoot on the floor with your legs outstretched in front of you. Raise your right leg slightly off the ground and draw large circles in the air using only your ankles. Put your foot back on the floor and repeat with your left ankle.

Sitting cross-legged stretches your thigh muscles

Hip circling

Lie flat on the floor with your arms by your sides, palms down. Bend both knees and cross your feet at the ankles. Then rotate your hips clockwise, making tiny circles with your lower back on the floor. Relax and then repeat the movement in the opposite direction.

Only raise your hips a little way up from the floor

Relax your jaw and concentrate on breathing evenly

Twisting and bending

Pregnancy hormones soften your ligaments in preparation for the birth; unfortunately they can also make you susceptible to strains and backache. Twisting and bending exercises help to strengthen key muscles, as well as to loosen up the pelvis in preparation for the birth. Getting down on all fours is an excellent way to ease backache, especially if you combine it with a few pelvic tilts.

Spinal twists
Lie on the floor with your arms stretched out and your legs together. Keeping your shoulders and arms flat on the ground, slowly bend your knees and turn them over to the left. At the same time, turn your head to the right. Then roll your knees to the right and your head to the left.

Spread your arms out at shoulder height

Gently rock your pelvis forwards arching your back

Stretch as far as you can but don't strain

Keep your head at this level; don't let it dip any lower

Keep your back straight; don't let it dip downwards

Pelvic tucks
Kneel on all fours with your knees about hip-width apart. Clench your buttock muscles and tuck in your pelvis so that your back arches up into a hump. Hold and then release. Repeat several times.

Forward bends
Place your feet shoulder-width apart, keeping them parallel. Slowly bend forwards from the hips, keeping your back straight. If you feel comfortable, extend the stretch by clasping your hands and raising them as far above your head as possible.

Squatting

There are many benefits to be derived from doing squatting exercises. Squatting cuts off some blood from the general circulation and so gives the heart a rest. It makes your joints, especially the pelvic ones, more flexible, stretches and strengthens the thighs and back muscles and relieves back pain. Squatting is a comfortable position to relax in and is a practical position for labour and delivery (*see p.181*). It may seem difficult at first but with practice it will become progressively easier.

Learning to squat
To begin with use a wall and pillows to prop yourself up. Place pillows on the floor. Stand with feet hip-width apart and your back against the wall. Slide down into a squatting position onto the pillows keeping your weight slightly forwards; you may not be able to put your heels on the floor at first.

Half squats
Hold onto something secure and place your left foot in front of your right. Point your left knee slightly outwards and slowly lower yourself to the floor, as far as you can go, keeping your bottom tucked in and your back straight. Stand up slowly and repeat with the other leg forwards.

Full squats
Keeping your back lengthened and straight, open out your legs and squat down as low as you can. Try to get your heels on the ground with the weight evenly distributed between heels and toes; don't worry if you have to raise your heels. Press your elbows against your thighs, to increase the stretch on the inner thighs and the pelvic area.

Keep your back as straight as possible

Press elbows into your knees to increase stretch

Sports activities

There are several sports that you can do as long as you take it gently and stop if you feel tired. Remember, if you're out of breath, your baby is deprived of oxygen. It is best not to go riding or skiing during pregnancy. Even if you're experienced you could fall. The risks are too great.

Walking

You can walk as much as you like – it's very good exercise. The main concern is that you walk under safe conditions.

Swimming

This is an excellent form of exercise during pregnancy and something you can generally continue doing until term. I swam two weeks before delivery with my second pregnancy, slowly and gently of course. Don't swim if the water is cold as you're more prone to cramp.

Cycling and dancing

Cycling is good exercise, but stop when your abdomen gets so large that it starts to affect your centre of gravity, as you might lose your balance. As long as you're not too energetic, you can dance throughout pregnancy. It's also a good way to practise some pelvic tilts.

Taking the weight
As well as improving your stamina, swimming supports your weight and helps you to relax.

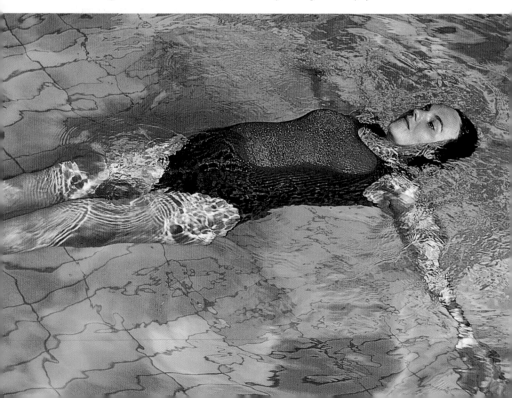

Travelling

Whether short or long distance, travelling is unlikely to do you any harm during pregnancy, but do use your common sense. Don't risk getting tired by taking long, unbroken journeys, particularly if you're on your own. Resist rough and jolting cross-country trips. Don't take travel sickness medication. Towards the end of your pregnancy, try to stay close to home, within easy reach of your doctor, midwife or the hospital.

Driving

You can drive until your size makes it hard to look over your shoulder, or until the steering wheel jams into your bump. For many women this occurs around the seventh month, for others there are no problems right to the end. It's illegal to stop wearing your seat belt just because you're pregnant.

Some women lose their ability to make quick responses and to concentrate without a break. If you notice this happening to you, it's unwise to drive for any distance. If you suffer backache during pregnancy, make sure you have a proper back support. Stop and get out of the car at least every 160km (100 miles) and walk around to rest your joints and keep the circulation going.

Trains

Going by train is probably the most relaxing way to travel on long journeys while you're pregnant. You can get up and stretch your legs whenever you want to and there's usually a toilet close by.

Flying

Travelling by air through time zones may be even more tiring during pregnancy because of your tendency to suffer fatigue.

Flying is not advisable after 36 weeks in a single pregnancy and after 32 weeks if you're expecting twins or more. Airlines have different policies about flying during pregnancy and may ask for a letter from a doctor or midwife confirming fitness to fly after you're 28 weeks pregnant. It's always a good idea to discuss your travel plans with your midwife first anyway.

If you do need to fly during pregnancy, bear the following points in mind.
- Ask the airline you're travelling with whether they offer any special seats or services such as early check-in for pregnant women.
- Get yourself some anti-embolism flight socks to wear on your journey.
- Always fasten your seatbelt below your abdomen.
- Avoid crossing your legs while seated in the plane.
- Pregnancy can also increase the risk of traveller's (deep vein) thrombosis so all pregnant women are advised to make sure they drink plenty of water during the flight. However, it's not generally recommended that pregnant women take low-dose aspirin before flying.
- Walk around the cabin at least once every hour to help your circulation and carry out some foot and leg exercises (*see p.125, 127*). Most airlines now provide details of these, especially if you're on a long-haul flight.

11 Looking good

In pregnancy, most women find that their skin improves and the legendary bloom appears as more blood flows under the skin, making them feel well and attractive. Exercise and a healthy diet, coupled with an awareness of the physical changes that occur in pregnancy, will contribute to you feeling happy with your changing shape and to giving you a good self-image. Taking care of your clothes, make-up and personal hygiene can also do a lot to boost morale. If you feel good, then you will probably look good too. You don't have to wear shapeless clothes; adapt your existing wardrobe for the first two trimesters.

What you wear

The increase in the circulation of blood throughout your body will cause you to sweat more and your vaginal secretions will also increase (*see p.152*). It's advisable to bathe or shower daily (but never to douche) and to wear, whenever possible, lightweight natural fibres that won't irritate your skin or make you feel hot and restricted. Even in cold weather you will be astonished at how warm you feel, so wear fewer and lighter clothes than usual for your own comfort.

Being pregnant is nothing to be ashamed of, and fashion designers now make maternity clothes that accentuate your bump attractively, using fashionable colours and flattering and comfortable fabrics. These can be worn right through your pregnancy to the birth, and beyond. Bear in mind, however, that your bust size

will increase, so figure-hugging tops may no longer fit comfortably. Also, avoid any garments that have a tight waistband or belt or fit closely around the thighs or crotch. Most women find that up to the fifth or sixth month they can get away with wearing their ordinary clothes, sometimes with a safety pin or a piece of Velcro to help the waistbands meet. Any garments with a drawstring or an elasticated waist can be adapted as your abdomen swells.

It's a wonderful boost to your morale to invest in one or two really smart or glamorous outfits. So that you have several months to enjoy them, don't wait until your pregnancy is too advanced before going out shopping. Remember that you don't have to buy maternity clothes. You should be able to find fashionable clothes to wear from the standard dress racks.

Your pregnancy wardrobe

Comfort is the watchword in pregnancy. Try to stay one step ahead of your growing size by buying clothes that are slightly too big so that you will always have something comfortable to wear.

- Look in the racks of maternity clothes for ideas and make a note of the way they allow for expansion with elasticated inserts and Velcro strips, for example. You can use the same techniques to adapt your existing wardrobe.
- Front hems on maternity dresses tend to be 2.5cm (1in) longer than usual, so if you make your own or buy a non-maternity dress, check you have the extra fabric in the hem.
- See if there is anything in your partner's wardrobe that you might borrow, for example a sweater or a shirt.
- Invest in a bump band, a stretchy fabric belt that allows you to wear your favourite jeans (undone).
- Loose-fitting jackets, shawls, fleeces and A-line coats are the best cover-ups.
- Choose natural fabrics such as cotton, wool or silk, which are more comfortable than synthetics in hot weather.
- Wear layers for comfort – a long shirt over a T-shirt, for example – so that if you get too hot you can easily remove the top layer.
- Big prints and wide stripes tend to make you look larger, whereas plain colours are more subtle.

Take pride in your appearance
Your pregnant shape is something to be proud of and for you to enjoy. See your swelling body as something beautiful, and don't ever worry about it.

- Stretch fabrics are comfortable, but avoid clingy materials.
- Try shopping online for maternity clothes; easier than trawling round the shops when you're pregnant.
- To cut the cost when buying a special outfit, visit shops that specialize in nearly new maternity clothes.
- On the beach wear a sarong or just a large T-shirt. Maternity swimwear is now both comfortable and stylish.
- A layered skirt with an elasticated or drawstring waistline can be worn under the armpits as a sundress, then pulled down and worn with a pretty top to make a versatile summer outfit.

Footwear in pregnancy

Whenever you can, go barefoot. Cotton or wool socks are often the most comfortable footwear, but tights are fine provided that they are large and stretchy enough, do not have a tight waistband, and the feet leave enough room for your toes to move freely. If you can tolerate wearing the waistband under the bump, ordinary tights will be comfortable throughout pregnancy, but during the third trimester you may need special maternity tights. Don't wear garters, stockings, or knee-high socks with elastic tops because these tend to make the blood stagnate in your legs.

Your feet and back are going to take the strain as you get heavier and your ligaments will soften and stretch. So, for the sake of foot comfort and posture, take care when choosing shoes. It's best to avoid high heels altogether as it's difficult to stand and walk well in them. In addition they can make you unstable.

Most of the time, at least, wear low-heeled shoes that are soft and comfortable.

Stylish close-fitting tops flatter your curves

Clothes for pregnancy
You don't need to buy a whole new wardrobe. A few special items supplemented with borrowed clothes will see you through.

A skirt with a stretchy waistband looks good and feels comfortable

If your feet swell, tight shoes may cut into your feet, but loose-fitting shoes can cause you to slip. Trainers are excellent, though laces may be difficult to tie later in pregnancy so opt for Velcro fastenings. For summer, wear adjustable sandals or canvas shoes that give if your feet swell.

Bras are important

You should always wear a bra in pregnancy because your breasts are becoming progressively larger and heavier, putting a strain on the supporting, non-elastic tissues. If you don't lift some of the weight from these ligaments, they will stretch and your breasts will sag permanently.

From the time your breasts start to get bigger, around weeks six to eight, wear a bra with a deep enough band under the cups, wide, comfortable straps and an adjustable fastening. If necessary, buy a bigger size as your breasts enlarge. If your breasts get very heavy, you may even want to wear a lightweight bra at night.

If you're planning to breast-feed, by about week 36 buy a special bra that will allow you to feed your baby easily. Babycare shops and department stores have a wide range of styles and sizes,

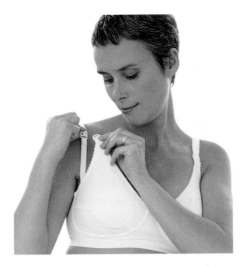

Feeding bra
This type of bra is suitable for the last stages of pregnancy and for breast-feeding. It gives plenty of support and the cups are easy to detach from the straps so that you can lower them for feeding.

but if you are an unusual shape or have a narrow or wide back, see an experienced corsetier or contact one of the childbirth organizations *(see p.242)*. You will be wearing this bra night and day for at least six weeks (buy at least two), so it needs to feel comfortable. You can buy some breast-pads now in readiness.

Skin and hair care

There are good reasons for the bloom that is said to appear on a woman's skin in pregnancy. The high level of hormones in your blood *(see p.92)* affects your skin, plumping it out, giving your face a smooth, velvety appearance. Added to this, your skin acquires a rosy glow because there's more blood circulating around your body. Most women find their skin improves noticeably, with dry skin becoming more supple, oily skin less shiny, and any tendency to spots disappearing – but the opposite can happen and you may have to adapt your whole beauty routine. Your face may become plumper, which tends to smooth out lines and wrinkles, making you look younger and healthier or, conversely, chubbier than before.

You may find that your skin itches more in pregnancy, particularly over your rounded abdomen. Rub any kind of oil into the skin. The oil itself may not make the difference, but the massage will certainly stimulate your blood vessels and ease the irritation.

If you have put on a lot of weight, especially on your thighs, your skin may chafe. Bathe frequently, dust the area with cornflour or talcum powder and keep it dry and cool. Wear cotton and avoid nylon tights. Calamine lotion is also soothing, but the only real prevention is to avoid gaining too much weight.

Chloasma

Any areas of your skin that are already pigmented, such as birthmarks, moles and freckles, can darken, especially in olive-skinned brunettes. Sunlight will intensify this so keep covered up or use a sun block. Occasionally brown patches (chloasma or the mask of pregnancy) appear on your face and neck. They are caused by the pregnancy hormones (see p.92) and are often noticed in women who have taken the contraceptive pill. Chloasma may be aggravated by a reaction to perfume, so test what you use. Don't try to bleach the marks out: cover them with concealer, topped with a thin layer of foundation. They will go within three months of delivery. Chloasma can be brought on by sunlight and it will get worse if exposed to the sun. If you can't avoid going out in the sun, use a strong sun block. Black women may develop patches of white skin on the face and neck. These too disappear after delivery.

Spider veins

These are broken blood vessels that resemble little red spiders. They appear on the face, particularly on the cheeks. They occur when a blood vessel dilates and tiny vessels grow from this central area. They are most noticeable in fair women but will have gone within two months of delivery.

Hair care

Many women notice a difference in their hair during pregnancy (see p.99). Some find their hair changes in quality, quantity and manageability. If your hair becomes difficult to manage, think about changing to a style that is easier to care for.

You can wash your hair as often as you like, but if you notice a change in your hair, use the correct shampoo for your new hair condition. Choose the mildest shampoo you can find. Use only one application of shampoo, massage gently to a lather, leave for 30 seconds and rinse off. Wash your hair in the shower or use the shower attachment when you take a bath so you don't put any strain on your back.

GENERAL SKIN CARE

- Use soaps as infrequently as possible on your face and body.
- Keep hand cream and lipsalve with you to use whenever necessary.
- If you wear make-up, don't stop now; make-up is good for your skin. It slows down the water loss from the skin, helping to rehydrate it.
- Use a bath oil in your bath water. It will leave a film of lubricating oil on your skin, helping to prevent water loss.

MAKE-UP CAMOUFLAGE TRICKS

If you wear make-up, a low-key, natural look is always flattering and makes the most of a fresh complexion. A style with startling details and bright colours won't do this. With your eye make-up, avoid hard colours – they will compete with the sparkle in your eyes – choose soft sludgy colours instead. There are always ways to camouflage any bad points, or at least to minimize their effects.

Wrinkles If your skin becomes drier than usual, fine lines, wrinkles and crow's-feet will look more obvious. Heavy foundations will accentuate them, so choose the finest texture foundation you can get, and use a fine, translucent powder.

High colour Increased blood supply can give you a permanently flushed look. To reduce this slightly, you can use anti-redness products, or apply a matt beige foundation that contains quite a lot of pigment but with no hint of pink. Stipple some onto the area of the cheeks where it's needed. Allow it to dry and then apply a thin layer of your usual foundation. Finish with a colourless powder. This is also good for concealing spider veins or any other red veins on your cheeks that become prominent.

Extra-greasy skin For greasy patches of skin, use a water-based moisturizer and oil-free foundation with translucent powder.

Extra-dry skin To deal with dry patches of skin, first apply a thin lotion that's absorbed by the skin within seconds, and on top apply a thicker kind that acts as a barrier to water loss. Covering the skin with a fine layer of suitable make-up also helps to slow down water loss. However, if your face is flaking, you won't be able to camouflage it, so abandon

all make-up and moisturize your skin thoroughly for a few days. Consult your doctor if the flakiness is accompanied by redness.

Puffiness It's most noticeable under the chin but can be camouflaged by shading a little brown blusher beneath the jaw-bone and either side of the neck. Apply blusher at the temples to draw attention to your eyes.

Dark circles Apply a thin layer of foundation. When dry, stipple over dark areas with an under-eye concealer. Leave for a couple of minutes, then cover with another thin layer of foundation, blending carefully. Dust with colourless powder.

Acne If you normally suffer from pimples or blackheads, you may find that they disappear. The fluctuation of hormones may, conversely, cause you to develop acne for the first time. This is different from ordinary acne, so don't treat it with the usual proprietary preparations. Talk to your doctor if you're worried – it will usually have vanished by the second trimester. To mask unsightly acne, stipple concealer or a extra foundation over the area with your fingers. Finish with foundation and then dust with colourless powder. Never squeeze a spot; this will spread germs into the deeper layers of the skin.

Make-up for pregnancy
Pick a foundation that is a shade paler than the skin on your neck and a translucent powder. Avoid pink blusher shades: those in the apricot range are more natural. Use a natural shade of lipstick to complete the effect.

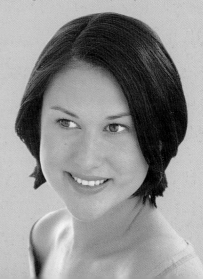

12 Rest and relaxation

During the first three months of pregnancy you're likely to feel very tired because, although your baby is still small, your body is having to cope with dramatic changes in hormone levels. By the second trimester your body will have adjusted and many women feel full of energy. In the third trimester, particularly the last six weeks, you're likely to feel quite exhausted again and need an extra two to four hours of rest every day. If it's hard to arrange a regular break, just take any chance you get to relax. If possible, lie down, even if you don't sleep. And, any time you're sitting down, put your feet up if you can. When you feel extremely tired, don't try to battle on, give in.

Sleep

During pregnancy it's essential to get an adequate amount of sleep, and you should always aim for at least eight hours a night. Paradoxically, though, however tired and even exhausted you feel at times, you may find you suffer from insomnia. When I was pregnant with my first baby, I well remember sitting out the early hours of dawn wondering why my fatigue didn't let me sleep. I didn't know the reason for my wakefulness then, but theories now advanced suggest that a mother's wakefulness is due to the ever-present metabolism of her baby.

The baby is growing and developing all the time in the womb, around the clock, so its metabolism doesn't slow down when evening comes – its engine keeps running at top speed. This means that the mother's body has constantly to fuel her baby with

food and oxygen, day and night, and her metabolism isn't allowed to slow down either. This is often reflected in the mother's inability to sleep.

Getting to sleep
Don't fight sleeplessness and become resentful – it will only make your insomnia worse – and don't take any sleeping pills without consulting your doctor. If you can't get to sleep or keep waking throughout the night and become increasingly restless lying in bed, try some of the following tips:
• Take the traditional remedy of a hot, milky drink before bedtime; this helps you to relax and wind down.
• Try having a warm bath before going to bed. This soothes both mind and body, making you feel sleepy and calm as well as relaxing your muscles. For many

women it acts like a knockout. Be careful, however, not to have too hot a bath before you go to bed as it may stimulate rather than relax you.

- Add aromatherapy preparations to your bath water: floral essences such as lavender, rose, geranium and chamomile are the best.
- Most pregnant women seem to need to spread themselves out when they sleep. If your bed is small it might be a good idea to invest in a larger one with a good supporting mattress fairly early in your pregnancy. A larger bed will also make it easier to achieve a comfortable position, propped up with several pillows, when you come to breast-feed.
- Avoid lying on your back (see p.144). Sleep on one side instead, in a position that you find comfortable. Get hold of some extra pillows or soft cushions and experiment with using them to make yourself more at ease. For example, when lying on your side, you might want to

When sleep is difficult
Make sure you're as comfortable as possible in bed, with extra pillows to support your legs and your bump in the later months.

put one pillow under your bump and another between your knees and thighs.

- Even if you have difficulty getting straight off to sleep, start going to bed earlier – you can read a book, which will help you to relax, or do some specific relaxation exercises (see p.140). Practise your deep breathing and concentrate on the new life inside you. Don't think of yourself as being lazy, just make sure that you get as much rest as you need.
- If you wake during the night, don't lie in bed fretting, get up and do something that you've been persistently putting off, or do some other useful task that could save you time next day. Make a cup of mild herb tea, such as rosehip, chamomile or peppermint, as these may help you settle to sleep again.
- Listen to some relaxing music, either on earphones in bed, or in another room.
- Make sure you don't become too hot during the night. Remember that during pregnancy your circulation increases, which can make you feel warmer. Keep your room well ventilated with the window and door open and, if necessary, change heavy duvets or blankets for lighter bedcovers.

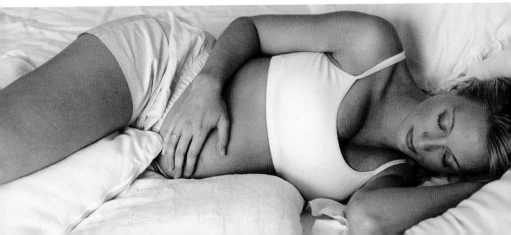

Learning how to relax

Impatience, irritability, an inability to concentrate and a loss of interest in sex are all signs of fatigue. Adequate rest can cure all of them. You can't always expect to get sufficient sleep at night, so you need to be alert to the possibilities of napping, or simply relaxing with your feet up, whenever the opportunity arises during the day. Long naps are not essential: five or ten minutes with your eyes closed and your feet up can be sufficiently refreshing. Something you'll never regret is learning a relaxation technique, which, once you're accustomed to using it, can recharge your batteries in a few minutes. If you want to control your body so that you can relax within 30 seconds, you might like to practise this method of instant relaxation or imagery training.

1 Arrange yourself comfortably.
2 Take a deep breath, hold for five seconds. Count to five slowly, then breathe out.
3 Tell all your muscles to relax.
4 Repeat this sequence two or three times until you're relaxed.
5 Imagine the most pleasant thought you can. An idyllic scene is ideal (see opposite). This helps you to use your imagination and to break down your mental blocks so that you can get more in touch with your body and learn to control it, which will be so useful during labour and birth.

Daytime rest
It's important to get enough rest, especially in the last trimester. If you find it difficult to sleep at night try to relax or have a catnap during the day.

PHYSICAL RELAXATION

This method involves giving orders in sequence to parts of your body to release the tension there. This is best learnt through tensing and then letting go. You will feel the difference in labour, when you should be able to relax most of the muscles in your body and let the uterus contract without the rest of your body tensing. Your partner can help you by touching you where he can see you're tensing up; you can respond to his touch by letting go.

It's best to practise this drill twice a day for 15–20 minutes if you can. Practise just before meals or an hour or more after eating.

1 Find a comfortable position lying on your back or propped up with cushions.

2 Close your eyes.

3 Think about your right hand; tense it for a moment, then let it go, palm upwards.

4 Tell your hand to feel heavy and warm, press your elbow into the floor or cushions, let it go.

5 Now work up through the right side of your body, through the forearm, the upper arm, into the shoulder. Raise your shoulder, let it go.

6 Repeat on the upper left side of your body. Both of your hands, arms and shoulders will now feel heavy and warm.

7 Roll your knees outwards, relaxing your hips, and press your lower back gently into the floor or cushions. Release and let the relaxation flow into your abdomen and your chest. Tell the muscles to feel heavy and warm.

8 Your breathing should start to slow down. If it doesn't, slow it down by counting to two between each breath.

9 Now relax your neck and jaw. With your lips together, drop your jaw with your tongue on the bottom of your mouth and your cheeks loose. Pay special attention to the muscles around your eyes and in your forehead – this will help to smooth away any frowns.

MENTAL RELAXATION

Once you've mastered the technique of muscle relaxation you can try relaxing your mind as described here.

1 Try clearing your mind of any stressful thoughts, anxiety or worry by breathing in and out slowly and regularly. Concentrate all your attention on your breathing actions, even saying to yourself very slowly "breathe in, hold, breathe out".

2 Let pleasant thoughts flow through your head and freely associate.

3 If any worrying thought recurs, prevent it from doing so by saying "no" under your breath or return to concentrating on your deep breathing.

4 With your eyes closed, imagine a tranquil scene such as a clear, blue sky or calm, blue sea. Always try to visualize something pleasant and blue because this has been found to be a particularly relaxing colour.

5 Think fairly hard about your breathing and become aware of it. Feel how it's slow and natural. Concentrate on each breath as you inhale and exhale. Listen to your breathing.

6 You should be feeling calm and restful by now – it might be helpful to repeat a soothing word or mantra such as love, peace or calm, or you may prefer a word with less symbolism such as breath, earth or laugh. Think of a word or even a calming sound like "ahhh" while you are breathing out.

7 Remind yourself to keep the muscles of your face, eyes and forehead relaxed and tell your forehead to feel cool.

It might help you to settle into your relaxation method if you adopt a starting routine. For example, if you repeat a mantra or drop your shoulders this can be the signal to the rest of your body to begin. Whenever you practise a relaxation method, make sure that you're breathing deeply, in the most controlled way (*see p.142*).

Breathing techniques

At antenatal classes you'll learn how to relax and master the various breathing techniques. You can use each one at different times during labour to help you to relax, conserve energy, control your body and pain, and calm yourself. This will give you more confidence during labour. Here are three basic levels that will help you.

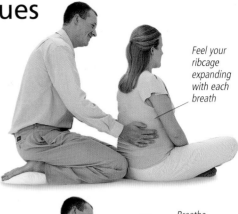

Feel your ribcage expanding with each breath

Deep breathing

When you breathe in, feel the lowermost part of your lungs fill with air and your lower ribcage expand outwards and upwards. Drop your shoulders. If someone places their hands on your lower back, you should be able to move their hands with your inhalation. It feels like the end of a sigh and is followed by a slow, deep exhalation. This is calming and ideal for the beginning and end of contractions.

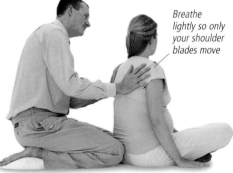

Breathe lightly so only your shoulder blades move

Light breathing

Aerate only the upper part of your lungs so that the top part of your chest and your shoulder blades lift and expand. Your breaths should be fast and short with your lips slightly apart. Draw the breath in through your throat. After ten or so light breaths you may need to take a deep breath – do so. This level of breathing is useful at the height of a contraction.

Featherlight breathing

The method I found most useful was panting. This is taking shallow breaths and resembles what you see and hear when a dog pants. Think of this as "pant, pant, blow". One of the times when you will be

Practise together
Practise breathing techniques with your partner, or whoever will be with you at the birth, so you can both learn the techniques to help you through labour.

asked to pant is during transition to stop you bearing down before the cervix is fully dilated (see p.178). When you're taking short, rapid, shallow breaths, your diaphragm is contracting and relaxing quickly and this prevents you from making a downward, concerted push. It's also useful to pant right through a painful contraction as you won't feel out of breath at the end. To stop yourself overbreathing, or hyperventilating, pant 10–15 times and then hold your breath for a count of five.

Massage

Physical contact is a source of comfort and solace at any time, but is especially helpful during pregnancy. Massage can be used as a means of relaxing you, and it also brings you and your partner closer together. It's very useful during the first stages of labour, not only for relieving any back pain but also for helping to reassure and soothe you.

Foot massage

With your partner well supported and comfortable, press with your thumbs on the soles and out to the edges of her feet. Firmness prevents you tickling her. Work from the heel up to the toes.

Massage the soles of her feet firmly

Stroking her brow

With your partner propped up against your chest, gently close her eyes and use your fingertips in a smooth outward movement, running your fingers out over her hair.

Gently stroke her temples with your fingers

Relieve back pain

With your partner lying on her side, feel for the base of the tail bone between the buttocks and press firmly with the heel of your hand. Make small circular movements to relieve back pain. Now move your hands down to her knees and smooth her thighs up to her buttocks.

Massage lower back with heel of your hand

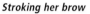

Comfortable positions

As your abdomen gets larger, sitting or lying in your usual positions can become uncomfortable. If you lie flat on your back for any length of time, especially in later pregnancy, the baby's weight presses down on major blood vessels running up your

Lying down
Lie on your side with the upper leg and arm bent up, and the other arm down by your side. You may find this position more comfortable if your upper leg is supported by one or more pillows.

Support your leg with cushions

Put pillows under your legs

Reclining position
If you find you can't rest lying on your side, prop yourself up in a reclining position with as many pillows as you need. This is very comfortable, especially in the later stages of pregnancy.

Putting your feet up
Lie on your back, with your head and back supported by cushions. Bend your legs and rest your feet on the wall. Straighten them out and let them fall as far apart as is comfortable.

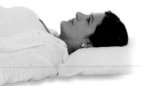

back. This can make you uncomfortable and dizzy as your blood pressure drops and it can aggravate haemorrhoids. For these reasons, it's not advisable to sleep, rest or exercise on your back. Carefully arranged pillows and floor cushions help, but don't lie with too many pillows under your head or your spine will be too curved. When sitting, don't cross your legs or bend them tightly as this may aggravate varicose veins. Try the positions below and always be aware of maintaining good posture.

Sitting up straight
This helps to strengthen the back muscles. A cushion in the small of your back may make you more comfortable, especially when you're driving. To rest at work, put your feet up level with your hips. Flex your feet from time to time to strengthen the backs of your calves.

Raise your feet to minimize swelling

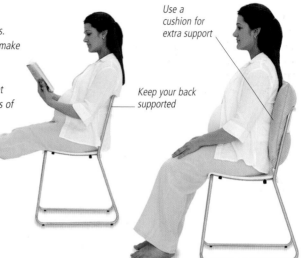

Use a cushion for extra support

Keep your back supported

Tailor sitting
Sitting cross-legged or with the soles of your feet together and your back straight opens up the groin and stretches the inner thighs. Gently press your thighs down to increase the stretch. This will help you to spread your thighs during childbirth.

Stretch inner thigh muscles by pressing on your knees

Legs apart
Sitting with your legs apart and your shoulders and back straight helps to stretch and strengthen the spine, inner thighs and groin. Flex your feet and feel the stretch along your thighs. Try to keep your shoulders relaxed.

13 Common complaints

Pregnancy is not an illness and most women have normal, healthy pregnancies that proceed without any problems. However, there is no denying that pregnancy can be an uncomfortable time.

COMPLAINT	CAUSES
Abdominal pain 2nd & 3rd trimester	Round ligament pain occurs during pregnancy when the ligaments supporting the uterus stretch.
Backache 1st, 2nd & 3rd trimester	Progesterone causes softening and stretching of the ligaments, most importantly in the pelvic joints. The ligaments supporting the spine also relax, which puts extra strain on the muscles and joints of the lower spine, pelvis and hips. Bad posture can make backache worse.
Bleeding gums 1st, 2nd & 3rd trimester	The gums thicken and soften due to the influence of the pregnancy hormones, which increases the body's blood supply. They swell, especially around the teeth, and food tends to collect in the hollows at the base of the teeth, allowing bacteria to grow and multiply, causing tooth decay and possibly gum infection (gingivitis).
Constipation 1st, 2nd & 3rd trimester	Progesterone causes relaxation of the muscles of the intestine and thus slows down bowel movements. Bowel contents tend to stagnate and dry out so that the stools become hard and painful to pass.
Cramps 3rd trimester	Thought to be a result of low levels of calcium in the blood. In rare cases it's due to a lack of salt in the diet.
Cravings 1st, 2nd & 3rd trimester	Thought to be related to high levels of progesterone.
Discomfort in bed 3rd trimester	Result of indigestion or heartburn (*see p.148*) or, when you lie down, the uterus presses on your diaphragm, stomach and ribcage.

Ailments in pregnancy

Many of the common complaints of pregnancy are irritating rather than real cause for concern, and being prepared for them is half the battle. Many of the aches and pains of pregnancy are due to a combination of tiredness and carrying around that extra weight. However, if you are at all worried about anything, don't be afraid to consult your doctor or midwife. He or she will be happy to discuss any anxieties that you have and will be pleased to be able to reassure you that all is well.

SYMPTOMS	TREATMENTS
Either felt as stabbing, cramp-like pain when you get up after sitting or lying for a time or a dragging pain on one side only.	None. Pain normally spasmodic so painkillers are not worthwhile. Apply a hot-water bottle to relax muscles. Do always seek advice if you suffer from prolonged or repeated abdominal pain at this time, just in case it's pre-term labour.
General ache across the lower back. Sacroiliac pain is classically across the top of the buttocks and extending down into them.	Good posture and exercises to strengthen the spine (*see p.126*) to make it more supple. Avoid very high heels; wear sensible shoes with a moderate heel. Have a good firm mattress on your bed. Avoid heavy lifting (*see p.119*). If the pain runs down your leg towards the foot, consult your doctor in case of a slipped disc. Try to avoid analgesics. Massage (*see p.143*) may help.
Gums are tender and bleed after brushing or eating hard foods. Gingivitis causes more bleeding than is normal after brushing.	Attention to oral hygiene is essential, with regular brushing of the teeth after food. Visit your dentist regularly but tell him you're pregnant as you should avoid X-rays at this time. There is no truth in the tale that the baby takes calcium from your teeth. Gingivitis should be reported at once to your dentist.
Infrequent hard stools. Pain in the lower abdomen.	Empty your bowels whenever your body tells you to. Have plenty of dietary fibre and fluid, preferably water. Exercise helps. Avoid strong laxatives and see your doctor if the problem persists.
Pain in the leg and foot, sufficiently painful to wake you. A hard knot of pain often followed for some hours by a general ache.	Very firm massage, possibly for several minutes; it also helps to flex the foot up and push into the heel (*see p.125*).
Strong desire for certain foods – prevents sleep and relaxation.	Indulge yourself, provided the foods aren't fattening, or cravings are for unsuitable substances (coal, for example).
Shortness of breath, acid regurgitation, soreness of ribs.	Try sitting up in bed with two or three extra pillows or try some of the positions on p.144. Get a firm bed and avoid heartburn (*see p.148*).

COMPLAINT	CAUSES
Fainting 1st & 3rd trimester	Pooling of the blood in the legs and feet when standing, together with the demands of the uterus for an increased blood supply, causes the brain to be relatively deprived of blood.
Flatulence 1st & 3rd trimester	Unwittingly swallowing air; also eating certain foods, e.g. pulses, fried foods and onions. In pregnancy the intestine is more sluggish and the wind may be more difficult to expel.
Frequent urination 1st & 3rd trimester	Early in pregnancy hormonal changes lead to differences in muscle tone that affect the bladder; also the growing uterus presses on the bladder, causing it to empty itself more frequently. Later in pregnancy the size of the uterus reduces the capacity of the bladder.
Haemorrhoids (piles) 2nd & 3rd trimester	The pressure of the baby's head in the pelvis in late pregnancy may obstruct the blood vessels in the rectum, impairing the return of blood from the pelvic organs and causing ballooning of the veins around the rectum. Anything that increases pressure in the abdomen, such as constipation, chronic coughing and lifting, will worsen haemorrhoids.
Heartburn 3rd trimester	The valve at the entrance to your stomach relaxes in pregnancy, allowing small amounts of acid to get into the oesophagus (the tube running from your mouth to your stomach).
Incontinence 3rd trimester	Pressure of the enlarging uterus on the bladder, thus reducing its capacity, and the inability of the pelvic floor muscles to stop leakage when you cough or laugh.
Insomnia 1st, 2nd & 3rd trimester	The general increase in your metabolism. The baby's metabolism doesn't distinguish between day and night so it may kick you at night. Also sweating and frequent urination may cause you to wake.
Itching 2nd & 3rd trimester	Itching is common and is caused by increased blood supply to the skin. If the itching becomes troublesome or generalized, particularly in the latter stages of pregnancy, it could be a potentially dangerous liver disorder, obstetric cholestasis. A blood test can confirm.
Morning sickness 1st trimester	Sudden high levels of hormones, particularly human chorionic gonadotrophin (hCG), the production of which closely parallels the time of nausea. It's not clear why it affects some women and not others. Diet before conception can predispose to nausea in early pregnancy, particularly a diet low in vitamins, minerals and carbohydrates. Tiredness also contributes, making nausea more severe, though it's not a cause.

SYMPTOMS	TREATMENTS
Dizziness, spinning, unsteadiness and need to sit or lie down	Avoid standing still for long periods of time. Don't jump up from sitting too suddenly and take care when getting out of a hot bath. Keep cool in hot weather. If you feel faintness coming on, lie down with your head flat and, if possible, raise your legs slightly.
Distension of the intestine, rumbling of the stomach, frequent passing of gas.	Try not to gulp air and avoid problem foods. Peppermint and hot drinks may help.
Urgent need to pass urine, even the smallest amounts, and at frequent intervals day and night.	Try reducing your liquid intake before going to bed. Later in pregnancy, try rocking backwards and forwards as you pass urine. This lessens pressure on the bladder and it may be more completely emptied. If you have pain or blood when passing urine, ask your doctor to check for urinary tract infection.
Itching, soreness, severe pain when passing stools, slight blood loss if the haemorrhoid is large and prolapses outside the rectum.	Prevent haemorrhoids with plenty of roughage, fluids and exercise, thus avoiding constipation. Try not to strain when you move your bowels. If you have haemorrhoids, keep the anal area clean to avoid irritation and apply an ice pack to soothe itching. Creams are safe to use. Minor haemorrhoids usually get better after delivery.
Burning sensation behind the breastbone sometimes associated with regurgitation of sour fluid.	Avoid the foods that give you trouble and don't eat a meal just before going to bed. Prop yourself up in bed and try a warm milk drink. Antacid medicines may be prescribed to help indigestion.
Leakage of urine under pressure within the abdomen, e.g. bending down, laughing.	Empty your bladder often, avoid heavy lifting and constipation. Do your pelvic floor exercises regularly (*see p.123*).
Difficulty going to sleep, or getting back to sleep after waking.	Wear light night clothes to avoid overheating. A hot milk drink or a warm bath (*see pp.138–139*) before bed may help. Try a drop of lavender oil in your bath. Sleeping pills are rarely prescribed.
Other symptoms of obstetric cholestasis may include dark urine, pale stools, jaundice.	If obstetric cholestasis is diagnosed, close monitoring under consultant care is essential. This may involve regular scans, cardiographs, blood tests and placental blood-flow scans.
Feelings of nausea at the sight or smell of food, or the smell of cigarette smoke. Occasionally accompanied by vomiting.	Eat little and often and avoid foods that make you nauseous. Don't get overtired, this will make your nausea worse. Try the diet ideas on page 114; suck peppermints or nibble dried fruits or dry biscuits; keep up your fluid intake. Talk to other pregnant women; if you know you're not the only one it may help. Your doctor will be loathe to prescribe any medication for you.

COMPLAINT	CAUSES
Nasal discomfort 1st, 2nd & 3rd trimester	Softening and thickening of the mucous membranes in the nose. Increase in blood supply to the lining of the nose due to high levels of pregnancy hormones. You may wake with a blocked nose in the morning. Rough blowing may rupture tiny blood vessels.
Oedema (swelling) 3rd trimester	Increase in fluid retained by your body and stagnation of fluid in the lower parts of your body and your fingers. Pressure of the uterus on the blood vessels that return blood from the lower parts of the body to the heart. Can be associated with pre-eclampsia (see p.160).
Pelvic discomfort 3rd trimester	The baby's head presses upon nerves, causing pain in the groin, particularly when the head is engaged in the pelvic cavity at the end of pregnancy.
Pigmentation 2nd & 3rd trimester	Increased production of melanocyte stimulating hormone (MSH) (see p.92). Made worse by exposure to strong sunlight.
Rashes 3rd trimester	Excess weight gain, poor hygiene and sweating in the folds of the skin.
Rib pain 3rd trimester	Costal margin pain results from the compression of the ribs as the uterus rises, the high position of the baby's head and excessive kicking by the baby.
Shortness of breath 3rd trimester	Pressure on the diaphragm prevents easy breathing. Lying down can also push the uterus and baby up against the diaphragm.
Stretchmarks 2nd & 3rd trimester	Depends on your skin type, and its elasticity. However, whatever your skin type, excess weight gain may cause stretchmarks (see p.98).
Sweating 2nd & 3rd trimester	Increased blood supply causes the blood vessels beneath the skin to dilate.

SYMPTOMS	TREATMENTS
Stuffiness in the nose, unexpected nosebleeds, congestion upon waking or runny nose.	Treat your nose gently. Avoid dry dusty atmospheres. Don't use a nasal spray without talking to your doctor. If you have a nose-bleed, apply gentle pressure to the soft part of your nose, just below the bridge. Lean forward slightly.
Swelling of the hands and ankles. Shoes feel tight. Your fingers may feel stiff in the morning.	Avoid standing, particularly in hot weather. Rest with your legs up, and rest at least once during the day. Avoid very salty foods. If you have severe oedema, your doctor may restrict your salt intake. Support stockings may help.
Pain in the groin and down the inside of the thighs, particularly bad after walking or exercising. Pins and needles spreading down the back of your legs.	Rest, avoid violent exercise and take an analgesic such as paracetamol, but consult your doctor first. Your doctor may check for movement in the symphysis pubis (see p.97).
Darkening around the nipple and areola, down the centre of the abdomen (linea nigra), deepening of pigmentation in freckles or birthmarks, mask across the face (butterfly mask) and down the sides (chloasma).	Use sunblock when you're out in strong sunshine. Don't ever bleach the skin. The pigmentation will fade within a few months of delivery.
Intertrigo is a red skin rash occurring where heavy folds of skin become irritated by sweat. Usually occurs under heavy breasts or in the groin area.	Keep the areas clean and apply a soothing lotion such as calamine. Dust with talcum powder after bathing or showering to make sure it's dry.
Soreness and tenderness, usually on the right side of your body. The pain is felt just below the breasts. It is severe when sitting up straight.	The pain will disappear as soon as the baby's head drops into the pelvic cavity prior to birth (or earlier in some women, especially those pregnant with their first child). Try not to compress the ribs: either sit up straight or lie down.
Shortness of breath on exertion.	Try to be less active. Rest in the day and go to bed early. If breathlessness is accompanied by chest pain or swelling, consult your doctor.
Silver marks on the skin of the thighs, abdomen and breasts.	Creams and ointments will have little to no effect. Eventually the marks will become smaller, narrower and a light silver colour, but they rarely disappear altogether. Make sure you do not put on too much weight too quickly.
Intense perspiration after light exertion or on waking at night.	Wear light cotton clothing and cotton underwear. Drink more to replace lost fluids.

COMPLAINT	CAUSES
Taste disturbances 1st, 2nd & 3rd trimester	Thought to be related to the pregnancy hormones.
Thrush 1st, 2nd & 3rd trimester	The yeast *Candida albicans* infects the vagina. Why it's more common in pregnancy is not known. The yeast can infect the baby's mouth at birth.
Tiredness 1st, 2nd & 3rd trimester	Sometimes because of worry, lack of sleep (see insomnia), poor nutrition, and towards the end of pregnancy the sheer burden of carrying around the unborn baby. Your body has to support both you and your baby.
Urinary tract infection (cystitis) 1st, 2nd & 3rd trimester	Slackening and relaxation of the muscle wall predisposes the bladder to infection at any time during pregnancy. The high level of progesterone is the cause. Symptoms may appear gradually over several weeks or months.
Vaginal discharge 1st, 2nd & 3rd trimester	Increased blood supply and softening and thickening of the mucous membranes result in a normal increase of mucoid discharge. Brown or yellow discharge could be cervical erosion, where the secretions increase due to overproduction by the cells at the neck of the womb. After sexual intercourse, spots of blood, not of a continuous nature, may appear. Heavy or smelly discharge may be a symptom of a sexually transmitted disease.
Varicose veins 1st, 2nd & 3rd trimester	A family history of varicose veins may mean that you develop them too. Near to term the baby's head can press down on the pelvic veins, causing blood to pool in the veins of the legs, and the result is ballooning of these veins. Standing for long periods of time will make swollen veins worse. Sitting with tightly crossed legs cuts off blood flow. Excess weight gain also causes the veins to dilate. Varicose veins on the vulva may result if the baby's head is interfering with the flow of blood there. The vulva then becomes swollen and congested.
Visual disturbances 1st, 2nd & 3rd trimester	Retention of fluid. If contact lenses feel different, this is because the eyeball has slightly changed shape with the increase in fluid.

SYMPTOMS	TREATMENTS
Often a metallic taste. Appreciation of the taste of certain foods alters. Coffee, alcohol and spicy foods, for example, become less palatable than before. Often increased liking for sugar and sweet things.	None.
Thick, white curdy discharge accompanied by intense itchiness. There can be some pain when passing urine.	Antifungals in the form of a pessary and a cream will be prescribed. They clear up the infection in two to three days. If the baby contracts the infection at delivery, a course of medicine will quickly clear it up. Don't wear tight or synthetic underwear during pregnancy.
Strong desire to sleep at odd times and needing more sleep at night. Legs ache and seem unable to carry you any further later in pregnancy.	Avoid overactivity. Sleep or rest whenever you can. Eat nutritious foods little and often to keep up your energy. Go to bed early. Get others to do the work.
Increased desire to pass urine accompanied by discomfort and pain. Urine may contain spots of blood. Dull discomfort in the lower abdomen.	Try to drink plenty of water. Cranberry juice may also help. See your doctor. Your urine will be tested and you will be given specific antibiotics to eradicate the infection.
Slight increase over normal of the clear, white discharge which does not cause soreness, pain or irritation. Discoloured or smelly discharge.	If the discharge is simply increased mucus, don't worry. Don't douche or use a vaginal deodorant. Wear cotton underwear and change it frequently, especially in warm weather. If the discharge is discoloured, smelly or includes spots of blood, check with your doctor.
Skin may be irritated or itchy at first, or there may be a dull aching pain. Then the veins start to appear as dark-purplish lines on the legs. A heavy feeling in the vulva.	Avoid standing around. Wear support tights; put them on before you get up in the morning after lying with your feet raised for a few minutes. Sleep with your feet on a pillow. Do exercises to improve circulation in your legs and feet (*see p.125*). For varicosity of the vulva, sleep with your bottom on a pillow or wear a sanitary pad firmly against the swollen part.
Long or short sightedness may develop. Contact lenses may be uncomfortable to wear.	If you notice anything different, go to an optician. Your prescription may change during pregnancy but may revert afterwards. If you wear contact lenses, tell the doctor or midwife at your antenatal clinic. You may have to stop wearing them during pregnancy.

14 Special-care pregnancies

Not every pregnancy is textbook and it's wrong to view some events, such as a multiple pregnancy, for example, as abnormal. You may have complications or unforeseen problems, but early medical intervention can help in most cases, provided the warning signs are recognized.

Pre-existing conditions

Anaemia

Pre-existing anaemia is no preclusion to pregnancy – about 20 per cent of women may be slightly anaemic before they conceive. The commonest form is iron-deficiency anaemia (when the haemoglobin level is less than 12.8g/100ml blood – *see p.71*) due to loss of blood at menstruation. Before you become pregnant, increase your intake of iron-rich foods and ask your doctor about iron supplements.

Diabetes

If you have diabetes, make sure your condition is well under control before conceiving, so that you've the best possible chance of a healthy baby and normal birth. You're likely to need more insulin during pregnancy and the doctor will monitor your drug requirements carefully as they may vary. You'll probably be seen more frequently than usual at the antenatal clinic and you should pay special attention to your diet. Some women are diagnosed as having gestational diabetes – diabetes that develops during pregnancy and generally

disappears soon after the birth. The risks of this are much lower and you rarely need insulin – often just cutting sugar out of your diet is enough.

Heart disease

Most women with heart disease have no problems in pregnancy, but they may need to take antibiotics to protect their heart valves while they are in labour. If you have a heart problem that carries a higher risk you will be warned by a cardiologist. Women with pacemakers or who have had heart surgery can usually undertake pregnancy safely.

Those who have suffered heart attacks or who have a muscle abnormality need advice from their cardiologist before conceiving. Having had a heart transplant is not a bar to becoming pregnant.

Hypertension

This is the medical term for high, or raised, blood pressure. Blood pressure is given as two figures, for example 120/70 *(see p.71)*. Doctors are more concerned about a rise in

INCOMPETENT CERVIX

Normally, the cervix remains closed so that the fetus is retained in the body of the uterus and doesn't fall into the vagina. If the cervical canal is open, it's described as an incompetent cervix. Although the reason is mostly unknown, cervical incompetence may be caused by late (after 12 weeks) surgical termination of a pregnancy or cone biopsy of the cervix, either of which may damage the muscle fibres that hold the cervix closed.

Usually an incompetent cervix remains undiagnosed until after the first miscarriage. The cervical canal starts to open by the 14th week and by the 20th week has dilated to about 2.5cm (1in), which is large enough for the bag of waters to bulge into the cervix and eventually break. There's usually a sudden loss of water, followed by a miscarriage with little pain. A special stitch is inserted around the cervix to tighten it; this is known as a Shirodkar McDonald, or purse-string suture. This can be performed before or during the next pregnancy. In the UK, the cervix is usually stitched during pregnancy, around the 14th week, under an epidural or general anaesthetic. This treatment has a high success rate and most pregnancies proceed normally. At about weeks 36–38, the stitch will be removed, labour usually beginning shortly afterwards either naturally or by induction. Some women do go to term.

the lower number, the diastolic pressure, which is a measure of the heart pumping when you are at rest.

If you know you have high blood pressure, talk to your doctor before becoming pregnant if you can. You may need to change your drugs and have your kidney function monitored. With proper care, there's no reason why you shouldn't have a normal pregnancy and labour. You may need to go into hospital early.

If you develop hypertension during pregnancy you may be monitored in an obstetric day unit as an outpatient, although a few women need to be admitted to hospital. It is sometimes necessary to deliver the baby early, possibly by Caesarean section, because of the effects of blood pressure on the mother or the baby.

Raised blood pressure in later pregnancy can be sign of pre-eclampsia, which is always taken seriously (see p.160).

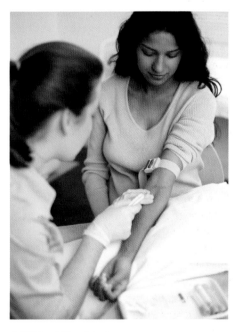

Additional blood tests
Blood tests will be carried out as part of your antenatal checks. However you may need extra blood tests if there are pre-existing conditions to monitor.

Antepartum haemorrhage

Placental abruption

If the placenta detaches itself from the wall of the uterus, it will bleed. The blood gradually builds up until it escapes round the membranes and through the cervix. Treatment may be bedrest and monitoring with ultrasound, followed by induction or possibly a Caesarean. Severe abruption is a medical emergency and will involve blood transfusions and an emergency Caesarean.

Placenta praevia

When the placenta is attached to the lower segment of the uterine wall, it is known as placenta praevia. If it lies partially or wholly over the cervix, it could be dangerous during labour as it could cause bleeding. Placenta praevia is detected by ultrasound scan. If there is any bleeding, you will be closely monitored and your baby delivered by elective Caesarean section.

Ectopic pregnancy

An ectopic pregnancy develops outside the womb, usually in the Fallopian tubes. It may cause abdominal pain because the tube is being stretched by the developing pregnancy or because of bleeding into the abdomen. Features that may increase the risk of ectopic pregnancy include a history of pelvic infection, use of a contraceptive coil (but not the Mirena) and a previous ectopic pregnancy. Women with a history of any of these are often seen early to check that the pregnancy is developing in the correct site. An ectopic pregnancy has to be ended by surgery or with drugs. Surgery may result in the loss of the affected tube, which may reduce fertility.

WARNING SIGNS OF PROBLEMS IN PREGNANCY

Contact the hospital maternity unit or your doctor immediately if you have any of the following symptoms, and while you're waiting, rest in bed. If you cannot contact the doctor, or he or she cannot come quickly, call an ambulance and alert the clinic that you're coming into hospital:

- Very severe nausea or vomiting several times within a short period, say two hours.
- Vaginal bleeding.
- Severe headache that doesn't go away, particularly in the second half of pregnancy.
- Severe abdominal pain.

- A fever of 37.8°C (100 °F) or over, regardless of the cause.
- A sudden reduction in the amount of urine you pass, for example if you don't urinate for 24 hours even though you're taking in normal quantities of fluid during that time.
- Rupture of the membranes.
- Absence of fetal movement for 24 hours from the 30th week of your pregnancy onwards.
- Sudden swelling of the ankles, feet, fingers and face.
- Sudden blurring of vision.

Multiple pregnancy

Twins are either identical – formed from a single egg – or non-identical when two eggs are fertilized. With identical twins, both babies usually share the placenta. Ultrasound will confirm the presence of twins or larger multiples from about the eighth week of pregnancy, but your doctor may be on the alert for twins anyway if:

• There are twins in your family.
• Your uterus is consistently bigger than your dates suggest.
• Two fetal hearts can be picked up with an electronic fetal stethoscope.
• As pregnancy progresses, two heads can be felt as well as multiple arms and legs.

If you're carrying twins, you will have special antenatal care with an emphasis on avoiding anaemia (see p.154). Expect to have regular blood pressure checks to make sure it doesn't rise, and take plenty of rest to keep your blood pressure low and damp down the sensitivity of the uterus to avoid premature labour.

A multiple pregnancy puts more pressure on your joints and on your digestive system. The large size of the uterus can also cause shortness of breath, piles, varicose veins and abdominal discomfort. At the first sign of any of these symptoms, ask your midwife or doctor for help, advice and treatment. You may suffer from more nausea in the first trimester but this is by no means the rule. You will probably have to have your babies in hospital because of the risk to the second baby if it isn't born straight after the first.

TWIN PRESENTATIONS

The most common presentation for twins is for both to be in the cephalic, or head down, position (*below left*) so delivery is usually straightforward. If one is breech and the other cephalic (*below right*), the cephalic baby is usually born first, stretching the birth canal so that the second one can be delivered easily. If both are breech, one baby is lying transversely (across the womb), or the babies are large, a Caesarean may be needed.

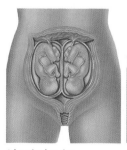

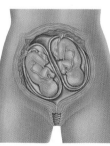

Identical twins
Developing from the fertilization of one egg that splits into separate cells, identical twins are always the same sex and look alike. They usually share a placenta but have their own cord and sac.

Non-identical twins
The result of two eggs that have been fertilized by two sperm, non-identical twins each have their own placenta and need be no more alike than any two children in the same family.

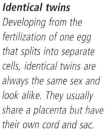

CEPHALIC   BREECH AND CEPHALIC

Miscarriage

A miscarriage happens when a pregnancy is lost before 24 weeks. It may be obvious that the pregnancy has ended because of bleeding and the spontaneous expulsion of the fetus, or the fetus might die in the womb with no outward signs of a problem. If, after the 24th week, a baby does not survive, it is called a stillbirth (see p.210).

Miscarriage is common and may affect as many as 20 per cent of all pregnancies. Most happen early in pregnancy (before 12 weeks) and most of these would never have survived, because of a developmental problem in the baby or a placenta that has failed to implant adequately. Many miscarriages occur before the woman knows she's pregnant. Miscarriages, especially those that occur after the first trimester, can also be caused by the following conditions:

- An incompetent cervix – the cervix sometimes fails to remain closed (see p.155). In the majority of cases, the cause is unknown.
- Abnormally shaped uterus that cannot sustain a pregnancy.
- An incompatible blood type (see p.160) that causes antibodies to your partner's

blood type to develop, resulting in the death of the fetus.
- Placental insufficiency – if the placenta is not functioning well or has not developed properly, it won't nourish the baby adequately.
- Maternal infections such as rubella.
- Uncontrolled diabetes or very severe high blood pressure.

What happens

Miscarriage is nearly always heralded by bleeding from the vagina, with or without abdominal pain. An early miscarriage may cause no more discomfort than a menstrual period without menstrual cramps. In some instances vaginal bleeding does not mean that a miscarriage will inevitably occur, but there's no way of you knowing, so you should always consult your doctor.

As far as a doctor is concerned, any bleeding during the first 24 weeks of pregnancy is considered to be a threatened miscarriage until it is proved otherwise. The bleeding may be light or it can be heavy, accompanied by the passage of mucus or not; there may be some backache and discomfort in the lower part of the abdomen. Doctors have come up with no better cause for a threatened miscarriage in the early stages than "hormone imbalance" or a "hormone insufficiency", which doesn't suppress the next period. If bleeding of this type occurs and the hormone levels remain low then miscarriage will almost certainly follow.

If a miscarriage threatens there's no evidence that rest makes any difference

---

IF A MISCARRIAGE THREATENS

- Call or visit your doctor.
- If you pass any clots or membranes, or the fetus and the placenta, collect them in a clean container and keep for the doctor to examine.
- Don't take any medicines or alcohol.
- Lie down flat if the bleeding seems heavy and keep your room cool.

and sadly there's nothing anyone can do to stop it. Many hospitals now have early pregnancy units where you may be offered a scan to check on your pregnancy. These units can usually support women in the early stages of pregnancy and deal with any problems that may occur. If, however, you have very heavy bleeding or you feel faint, go to the nearest emergency department immediately.

If you do have a miscarriage the unit may suggest one of three options: managing it medically with tablets or pessaries, waiting for nature to take its course, or having your uterus emptied under anaesthetic (a D&C or ERPC or evacuation), usually as a day procedure.

Emotional effects

Miscarriage at any time, but particularly one that occurs during the second trimester of pregnancy, has a profound psychological effect on a woman. This is due not only to the loss of the baby and the wide range of emotions resulting from that, but also because of the sudden withdrawal of pregnancy hormones without the reward of having a baby. There are many fears – about your own inadequacy, that you may never be able to carry another baby, that your fertility may be permanently affected, that you had an abnormal baby this time and that you could have another next time.

I also think that there is a feeling of real bereavement. I suffered a miscarriage myself at 14 weeks and was actually shown the fetus, which was well enough formed to distinguish that it was a boy. For about six weeks afterwards I found myself in a deeply depressed state.

TYPES OF MISCARRIAGE

Threatened miscarriage A miscarriage is possible but not inevitable; there is bleeding from the vagina, rarely accompanied by pain.
Inevitable miscarriage Vaginal bleeding is accompanied by pain due to the uterus contracting. If on internal examination the cervix is dilated, virtually nothing can prevent the expulsion of the fetus. The miscarriage may be complete or incomplete.
Complete miscarriage The fetus and placenta have been expelled from the uterus.
Incomplete miscarriage The fetus has been lost but some of the products of conception, such as parts of the placenta, are still in the uterus and may have to be removed surgically.
Recurrent miscarriage A miscarriage has occurred on more than one occasion, for different reasons and at different stages of the pregnancy.
Missed miscarriage The fetus is no longer alive but is still in the uterus. The fetus will be expelled by the uterus eventually. A missed miscarriage may be diagnosed at a routine scan.

After a miscarriage your emotions need careful handling, because they may be complicated by feelings of guilt and blame. Try to talk about your feelings with your partner and with your doctor.

The next pregnancy

When you start the next pregnancy is a matter of choice and planning, but take as much time as you need. From a medical point of view, sexual relations can begin as soon as the bleeding has stopped, and my advice has always been to try to start a pregnancy as soon as you both feel ready.

Pre-eclampsia

Also known as pre-eclamptic toxaemia (PET), pre-eclampsia is a potentially serious condition that can affect as many as one in ten women, especially first-time mothers and women carrying more than one baby.

SIGNS OF PRE-ECLAMPSIA

Pre-eclampsia does not have any outward symptoms, and many women who are diagnosed as having it are surprised and frustrated, as they may feel perfectly well in themselves. Staff at antenatal checks will be alerted to its presence if:
• You have raised blood pressure, especially if it's consistent over a couple of weeks. An increase that would ordinarily be insignificant may be considered abnormal during pregnancy.
• Protein is detected in your urine – it signals potential damage to the kidneys.
• There is swelling (oedema) to the feet, ankles or hands, or puffiness in the neck and eyes.
• You suddenly gain weight excessively.

This is a condition that is unique to pregnancy, and it can start at any time during the second half.

It's not known precisely what causes the condition, but it does tend to run in families. It arises in the placenta so the baby may grow more slowly than normal. The pregnancy cannot be restored to normal once you have pre-eclampsia, so your condition and that of your baby will be monitored closely, probably in hospital – possibly in a day unit. In this way delivery can be arranged quickly before serious complications arise. For almost every mother, delivery of her baby reverses the condition, although your blood pressure may remain raised for up to six weeks after the birth, requiring treatment to bring it under control. If your pre-eclampsia was so severe that you were in danger of seizures, leaving hospital early isn't recommended as the risk of having a seizure remains for up to five days after the birth of the baby.

Rhesus incompatibility

The blood sample taken at your first antenatal visit will reveal your blood group (see p.73). As well as this, the test will indicate your Rhesus (Rh) grouping, either positive or negative. Rhesus negativity is much less common than Rhesus positivity – only about 20 per cent of the population is Rhesus negative. If your partner has Rhesus-positive blood the chances are that you'll carry a Rhesus-positive baby.

As a Rhesus-negative person, your immune system will perceive Rhesus-positive blood as foreign, and if you're exposed to it, for instance by a transfusion, you will develop antibodies to Rhesus-positive blood cells that will kill them.

If you have a Rhesus-positive baby and blood cells from the baby pass into your circulatory system, your body will try to destroy them with Rhesus-positive antibodies.

With your first baby there is little danger because you are being exposed to Rhesus-positive blood cells probably for the first time and the level of Rhesus antibodies will be low or even absent. Blood cells may, however, pass between you and the baby during delivery, vaginal bleeding, abdominal injury, amniocentesis, CVS and external cephalic version (turning a baby who is in the breech position – *see p.203*), which can cause your blood to make antibodies.

Danger during subsequent pregnancies can also be insignificant because antibodies may never be formed in large enough quantities. However, at various points during your antenatal care doctors will take the precaution of finding out what level of antibodies is present in your blood. It's known that a certain level of antibodies may damage the developing baby. This level, however, is reached in less than ten per cent of women who are Rhesus negative. Don't be despondent, therefore, if the doctor tells you that you have Rhesus-negative blood. In practical terms all it may mean is that you get extra-special medical care.

Beating Rhesus incompatibility

Rhesus incompatibility in pregnancy is becoming less and less common as the condition is better understood. After any of the risk episodes listed, you will be given anti-Rhesus globulin (Anti-D). It may also be given twice routinely to pregnant women who are Rhesus negative but have no antibodies, to make sure your baby is safe from Rhesus incompatibility whatever the circumstances.

If you have antibodies already and they exceed a critical level you will probably be referred to a specialist unit where your baby will be assessed.

HOW RH INCOMPATIBILITY OCCURS

In a first pregnancy there is rarely a problem as the maternal and fetal bloodstreams do not mix during the pregnancy. If some of the baby's Rhesus-positive blood cells escape into the maternal blood during delivery, they may react to form Rhesus antibodies. In subsequent pregnancies, these Rhesus antibodies may cross the placenta and damage the baby's blood if it is Rhesus positive.

KEY – *Rhesus negative* + *Rhesus positive* ▲ *Rhesus antibodies*

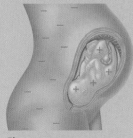

First pregnancy
Maternal and fetal blood systems are completely separate throughout the pregnancy.

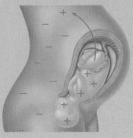

Delivery
Some of the baby's blood leaks into the mother's blood, which generates Rhesus antibodies.

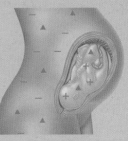

Subsequent pregnancy
Rhesus antibodies in the mother's system can affect a Rhesus-positive baby's blood.

15 Preparing for the birth

By the 36th week of your pregnancy, you will probably have given up work and be taking things a little more slowly. You may feel frustrated and bored, you may welcome the rest from your work and the travelling, or you may feel energized and want to spring-clean the house. This is the time to check that everything is ready for the new arrival and to prepare yourself, your partner and your other children for the birth.

Organizing your home

There are many things you can do to prepare yourself and the household to cover your day-to-day routine and make life easier for you after the baby is born.

- Start to neglect certain parts of your domestic life. Allow the non-essentials to slide and don't worry about them.
- Stop doing any housework that involves hard physical effort.
- Make sure that your family realizes that you can't dash around as you used to. Get others to help with errands.
- Try not to worry about things that don't matter. The highest priority is the baby that is growing inside you.
- Sound out a reliable neighbour who will help in emergencies.
- If you've a freezer, stock it with staple foods that freeze well, such as bread, butter, soups, casseroles and vegetables.
- Stock up your cupboards with tinned and dried foods and basic essentials such as washing powder, toilet rolls and disposable or reusable nappies.

Getting the baby's room ready

If you've enough space, you can give your baby a separate room and make it into a nursery, but this isn't absolutely necessary – your baby's space can be a corner of a larger room. Even if you've planned a separate nursery for your baby, you'll probably find you hardly use it in the early weeks – it's recommended that your baby sleeps in the same room as you for the first six months, particularly at night, to help avoid SIDS. You will probably want to keep him close by you in his cot or Moses basket the rest of the time as well.

After these first few weeks, it is ideal to have a room that is equipped for all your baby's routines, such as feeding, bathing, changing, dressing and playing. However, you don't need to go to a lot of expense. Most baby equipment can be purchased second-hand. Look around in local papers and shop windows or at your baby clinic; friends often lend equipment too.

Preparing a nursery
*Once you have the essential items
like a cot and bedding, you can
enjoy decorating the nursery –
you'll have little time once your
baby is born.*

What you need for your baby

It's helpful to start thinking about what you need for your baby quite early in your pregnancy, particularly if you're planning any structural changes to your home.

Baby equipment

- **Crib and cot** – a crib is a luxury for the first few months. Your baby can just as easily sleep in a Moses basket. A tiny baby can sleep in a full-size cot provided you do not impede air circulation with a cot bumper and you lie him down "feet to foot" – with his feet touching the foot of the cot so that he cannot wriggle down under the blankets.
- **Moses basket** – this can be useful for up to six months depending on the size and vigour of your baby. It can be used as an alternative crib.
- A rear-facing **baby car seat** that can be secured to the front or back seat of the car. Do not use a baby seat in the front seat of a car with airbags.

ESSENTIAL BABY CLOTHING

- Six stretch suits – you may be showered with tiny clothes for the baby. The first size only lasts about six weeks, but you will need several because of frequent soiling.
- Two nightdresses – these make nappy changing easy in the early days.
- Four vests – envelope necks are best.
- Two cardigans or jumpers – avoid lacy patterns that are impractical as little fingers get caught in the holes.
- Two pairs cotton socks or bootees.
- One hat or sunhat.

- For the crib or cot, choose a firm, flat **mattress with a waterproof cover**. Babies should never have pillows as they might suffocate in the fabric covers.
- **Towelling fitted sheets** or **flannelette** for warmth – at least four or five.
- Only use **cotton cellular blankets**; wool may make him too hot. Duvets should not be used for babies under 12 months.
- **Muslin squares** for catching possets and protecting your clothing during burping sessions. They can also be stretched across the cot under the baby's head to catch any posset and protect the sheet.
- **Nappies** – you can choose reusable nappies or disposables, or a combination. Studies have shown that when the cost of reusable nappies, nappy cleansing solution and electricity for the washing machine are added up, disposables are not that much more expensive. Resuables are better for the environment though. You could try disposables for the first few weeks to give yourself a break from the washing. If you use fabric nappies, buy at least two dozen shaped nappies with Velcro fastenings or terry towelling squares with separate nappy pins/ grippers. You will also need two plastic buckets with lids, and cleansing solution.
- **Nappy liners** – disposable liners are useful inside fabric nappies as they can contain stools and thus reduce staining.
- At least six pairs of **plastic pants** if you're using fabric nappies. They quickly become brittle and crack. So buy the best quality and try to wash them by hand.
- **Baby bath** – this is useful as it means

you can bath your baby in the warmest place, not necessarily in the bathroom. It's best to wait till your baby is about four months old before you start using the big bath.

- **Plastic changing mat**.
- Two soft new **towels** for the baby's use – your own towels will feel like sandpaper against your new baby's perfect skin. Towels with hoods are cosy.
- **Baby bath solution**.
- **Natural sponge** or soft facecloths.
- **Cotton wool**.
- **Vaseline, cleansing lotion,** and **baby wipes** for changing time.
- **Olive oil** for flaky skin.
- **Blunt-ended scissors**.
- A **changing bag** – it unfolds to reveal a waterproof area for changing the baby and has pockets all around that hold nappies, change of clothes, cleansing lotion and nappy pins/grippers. It can then be rolled up and slung over your shoulder after the change.
- **Pram** or **pushchair** – you will have to do a lot of research here to decide on your needs. If you have a car and drive everywhere, a pram with collapsible frame is perfect. If you travel on public transport, a pushchair that collapses easily and adjusts to the horizontal position is ideal. There are so many designs now, so shop around and ask other parents.
- **Sling and back-pack** – the sling is for the first six months or so, depending on the weight of the baby, but a back-pack for an older baby can also be useful, especially for a baby who has become accustomed to being carried around.
- **Feeding equipment** if you're not breast-

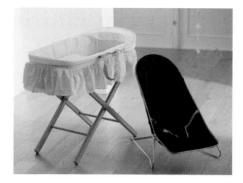

Baby equipment
A Moses basket is a simple and lightweight bed for a newborn. A bouncing baby chair with a back support is also useful for young babies before they can sit up.

feeding, or if you express milk for someone else to feed to your baby.
- A **bouncing cradle** – in this reclining seat your baby can be partly propped up and can watch you moving around the room.

Arranging a nursery

See that all the surfaces in the nursery are hygienic and easy to wipe clean. Make sure that there is plenty of storage space, especially around the changing area. Open shelves for storage mean that it is easy to reach your baby's belongings. Floor-level cupboards will need baby safety locks later on when your baby becomes more mobile and inquisitive.

Fit a dimmer switch for night feeds. Heat control is also important; the temperature should be constant at around 18–20°C (65–68°F), so your baby is neither too hot nor too cold. For your comfort you'll need a low feeding chair and a table. It may be a bit of a luxury, but if it's possible, install a small sink with running water in the room.

Getting ready for the birth

The hospital or your midwife will give you a list of the items you will need to take with you for the birth. If you're having your baby at home, you will need to prepare a room for the birth.

Preparing for a home birth

There are some useful ways you can make your home birth comfortable for yourself and convenient for the midwife.

- Make sure your bed is firm so that you have something to push against and you can avoid getting a puddle of amniotic fluid under your hips. If necessary, put a board under the mattress. You may decide not to use the bed but have it ready so that all your options are open.
- The most convenient way to make the bed is as follows. Make it up with fresh sheets. Put on a plastic sheet (an old shower curtain will do) and cover with clean old linens. In this way the old sheets and plastic can be taken off after the birth, leaving you in a freshly made bed.
- Provide polythene sheeting to protect furniture and flooring in the room in which you're going to give birth.
- Prepare a work area, such as a table top or a dressing-table, that is within easy reach of the bed for supplies.
- The maternity pack provided by the midwife before the birth will contain many of the items necessary for the birth. Check with your midwife to see if she will bring a sterile sheet.
- Clear a large area of the room if you plan to have a mobile labour. Have some freshly washed sheets nearby in case you prefer to deliver on the floor when the time comes.
- To prepare yourself you should have a bath, or a shower to avoid infection if the waters have broken. Otherwise, wash your hands to beyond the wrists, your thighs 30cm (12in) down either side and the pubic area with antiseptic

Advance preparations
Make a list of everything you need for your delivery. Prepare it in advance and ensure your birth partner knows where to find it.

soap, and dry with a clean towel, sterile cloth or gauze pad.

- Have ready a clean nightdress, sanitary pads and underpants for yourself, and a cotton cellular blanket, a disposable nappy and a nightdress or stretch suit for the baby. Prepare a Moses basket or cot with the baby's bedding in place.

Extra items for home birth

As well as the items shown and the equipment provided by your midwife, you may also like to have the following items to hand:

- Hot-water bottle for comfort during labour and for soothing afterpains.
- Some nourishing, easily digested snacks and drinks.
- Hand mirror to help you see the birth.
- Camera with plenty of batteries and film or an empty memory card.
- Presents for siblings from the baby.
- A supply of disposable knickers.

What to take to hospital

Several weeks before your baby is due, pack your hospital case with all the things you will need for your stay there. Ask the hospital if they provide a clothes list. Few hospitals provide nappies or baby clothes during your stay, though most provide bedding. You may find that your partner has to fetch and carry clean and soiled clothing during your stay, and then will have to bring in day clothes for you and something for the baby to wear when you're discharged from hospital. Remember to set aside loose-fitting clothes. Your breasts will have increased greatly in size when your milk comes in (see p.221) and your abdomen won't have gone down yet.

USEFUL ITEMS FOR HOSPITAL

For you
- Two to three front-opening nightdresses.
- Two to three maternity bras and breast pads.
- Dressing gown and slippers.
- Four pairs of pants; disposable are useful.
- Sanitary towels – get the most absorbent you can find.
- Toilet bag and contents – soap, toothbrush, toothpaste, cleanser, moisturizer and shampoo.
- Hair brush, two towels, two facecloths.
- Tissues or a soft toilet roll.
- Make-up and mirror.

For the baby
- A packet newborn-size disposable nappies.
- Three vests.
- Three stretch suits or nighties.
- Cotton cellular blanket.

Aids for partner to bring
For hospital delivery your partner or birth assistant will also need to pack a small bag with the following items:
- A small natural sponge to moisten your mouth.
- Lipsalve or Vaseline to prevent your lips becoming chapped.
- Frozen picnic freezing pack or hot-water bottle to soothe backache.
- A bottle of diluted fruit juice or water for you to sip during labour.
- Drinks and sandwiches for you in case either of you want something after delivery.
- Books, playing cards, Scrabble, jigsaws, music player to occupy you both while you're waiting between contractions.
- Leg warmers or thick socks if you start to shiver during the later stages (see p.178).
- Facecloth to mop your face if you're too hot.
- Coins or phone card for the hospital phonebox.

Involving your other children

If you have a family, every member should be involved in your pregnancy. Children should be told about what is going on and how the pregnancy is progressing, according to their age and how much information they can absorb and understand. Even a very young child will notice that your shape is changing and will want to know why. Give an honest and accurate answer and let your child feel the baby kicking inside you. If your child or children are old enough, put a chart up on the wall of what happens to you and the baby in pregnancy and follow it through as your pregnancy progresses.

If you're having a home birth, decide whether you want your children to be with you. It is sensible not to restrict the child and if he follows your pregnancy through, the experience will be an enlightening one. Don't be surprised, though, if he gets bored at the time and wants to go off and play. There needs to be someone responsible there, besides your partner, to take care of him during the labour.

Run through everything with him, especially the fact that it is a bit painful and you are likely to call out, otherwise he may be frightened. You should also prepare him for the birth of the placenta, which is often the bloodiest part. Warn him that you won't be able to answer his questions because you'll

be busy and that if the midwife asks him to leave the room at any stage, he must do as she says and not hesitate.

Make arrangements

If you're going into hospital, explain to your child what is going to happen and what arrangements will be made, as long as he is old enough to understand. Even if you will be in hospital for a short time, say 24–48 hours, you'll need someone to take care of your child. If you possibly can, ask someone he knows well to come and look after him in his own home so that his normal routine isn't disrupted too much and he has all his familiar objects around him. If this isn't possible and he has to be looked after in someone else's home, make

Keeping your children involved
Chart the progress of your pregnancy with your older children and involve them so they understand what is happening.

sure it's somewhere he knows well and where he has spent the night more than once well before the birth – if you have a long labour it could be 18–24 hours before you or your partner are able to collect him.

Make sure that your child knows exactly how long you're likely to be apart. Prepare him in other ways by pointing out small babies to him; show him pictures of his own babyhood and relate this to the coming arrival. Buy him a doll of his own so that he feels he has a baby too. It helps too if your partner spends extra time with your child, particularly with usual routines like bathing, feeding and storytelling.

If your child is old enough to understand, rehearse what is going to happen so that he becomes familiar with the future events. It is surprise that will upset him. Make a timetable of what you will do when labour starts. If you go over this together several times he will feel happy and secure in the knowledge that you're taking special care of him.

COUNTDOWN FOR LABOUR

Home birth
1 Ring the midwife.
2 Ring your partner or birth assistant.
3 Contact whoever is caring for your other children and alert them.
4 Make yourself a hot drink.
5 Check that the room is ready.
6 Have a warm bath or shower.

Hospital birth
1 Ring the hospital, then call an ambulance or taxi if you're not being driven in by your partner or a friend. Don't drive yourself.
2 Ring your partner or birth assistant.
3 Alert whoever is caring for your children that you're going in.
4 Make yourself a hot drink.
5 Collect together your handbag, coat and your packed bag.
6 Rest and wait for your partner or the ambulance. If someone is driving you to the hospital, you should know how to get there and how long it will take. Plot an alternative route in case the traffic is heavy or you find the road blocked for some reason. Whenever possible, choose well-made roads with no speed bumps, so that your journey will be comfortable. Find out from the hospital which entrance you should use, during the day and night, to get you to the ward by the most direct route. Make sure you and the driver are thoroughly familiar with all this information and, if it puts your mind at rest, do a trial run.

Signs of labour
In the week or two before you actually go into labour you may experience signs that something is about to happen.
1 You feel a "lightening" or engagement, when the baby's head drops into the pelvis.
2 The baby's engagement causes an increase in pressure on your bladder and you will find that you want to pass urine more frequently again.
3 Braxton Hicks contractions become more frequent and may get stronger.
4 Often vaginal secretions increase a day or so before labour starts. If it's your first baby you may have a "show" (*see p.171–172*) as much as two weeks before labour.
5 Slight weight loss in the last week.
6 Some women experience a nesting instinct, wanting to clean the house.

16 Labour and birth

This is the point to which all your preparations have been leading. While it's unrealistic to expect the birth to be pain-free, you can hope for it to be relaxed and happy. It'll help if everything and everyone around you are familiar. And you'll be calmer if you understand what's happening and feel confident that you can control your body during the delivery. If you learn about labour and practise the exercises and breathing techniques, you should feel less pain and be alert to the joy and beauty of giving birth.

Labour

Your labour can be divided into well-defined stages. There is a stage before it begins, sometimes called pre-labour. The first labour stage is divided into two; the early phase is when you start going into labour and when contractions may be short, irregular and not too painful. This culminates in the late first stage of labour and a transition to when your contractions become regular, more frequent and painful, resulting in full dilatation of the cervix. The second stage of labour is when you push the baby through the birth canal and it ends with the birth of your baby. Labour is not complete until you have gone through the third stage, which is delivery of the placenta (afterbirth).

Every woman feels the pain of contractions differently, but in early labour they may be similar to menstrual cramps and sometimes they're confined to mild backache. The kind of labour that proceeds well into the first stage with nothing more than gradually worsening backache is often called a backache labour (see p.174).

Pain in labour

Very often a contraction feels like a wave of discomfort across your abdomen that reaches a crescendo for a few seconds and then diminishes. At the same time you will feel a hardening and tightening of the uterine muscle, which is held at the peak of its intensity for a few seconds and then begins to relax again. You will have no control over your contractions – they are "involuntary" – although your state of mind during labour can have a deep effect on contractions, and can make them feel more or less painful.

Most women assume that contractions will get longer, more frequent and stronger in a steady pattern. This is not so; don't be disturbed if your contractions seem to vary.

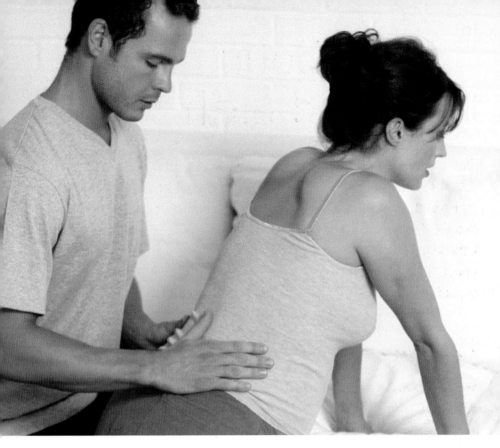

Loving support
Some women find that touching and stroking at any time during labour are immensely helpful.

It is absolutely normal for a strong contraction, for example, to be followed by a weaker one that doesn't last quite as long. It is also normal for contractions to follow one another relentlessly – this is more likely if labour has been induced and then is kept going with an intravenous drip (*see pp.197–199*).

Onset of labour

Most people think the onset of labour will be very clear: pains will come, contractions will start and you'll know it has started. In reality, it often isn't clear at all.

Three things might happen once it begins, although they don't necessarily mean that birth is imminent.

- The blood-tinged, gelatinous plug of mucus that has blocked the cervical canal may become dislodged during the early first stage of labour (although this can happen as much as two weeks before labour starts), and it always precedes

LENGTH OF LABOUR

Labour is usually longest with a first baby, an average 12–14 hours. Thereafter labour lasts an average seven hours. In general, the lighter the contractions, the longer the labour will be. A fast labour tends to start with long, slow contractions and proceeds in the same way.

rupture of the membranes. It is sometimes called the "show" and means that the cervix is beginning to stretch.

• Your membranes may rupture at any time up to the delivery. Leakage of the amniotic fluid varies from a gush to a slight dribble that can be stemmed by wearing a sanitary pad. There is no pain when the membranes rupture and the flow depends on the site and size of the break and whether or not the baby's head is plugging the hole. If your membranes rupture you should contact the midwife or the hospital immediately.

THE PRESENTATION

The presenting part of your baby is the part that will be born first. Most babies lie in a well-flexed (curled-up) position with the chin resting on the chest (*below right*). The way a baby presents can affect labour and birth; a posterior presentation (*below left*) can lead to an erratic backache labour (*see p.174*). If the face is presenting, labour may be slower and the baby's features may be slightly swollen for about 24 hours.

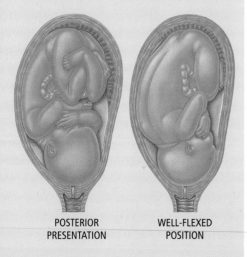

POSTERIOR
PRESENTATION

WELL-FLEXED
POSITION

• You may feel a dull backache or, if you had Braxton Hicks contractions during the third trimester, you may mistake the early contractions of labour for stronger Braxton Hicks. Severe Braxton Hicks can be mistaken for labour, however, and this is known as a "false labour". Time these early contractions over an hour and if they get closer together and longer in duration, you're probably in labour. The intervals between contractions – once it's established that you're in labour – are timed from the end of one to the beginning of the next. The contractions tend to be 30–60 seconds long at first, building up gradually to 75 seconds during the most active phase of labour.

Admission to hospital

When you reach the hospital labour ward the midwife will prepare you for the birth. Your birth attendant can stay with you while she does this.

• She will consult your notes and ask you about the labour so far – whether your "waters" have gone, how frequently the contractions are coming and whether or not you have moved your bowels.

• She will ask you to change into the loose clothes you have brought with you to wear for the labour and birth.

• You will be examined; the midwife will palpate your abdomen to feel the baby's position, she will listen to the fetal heartbeat, take your blood pressure, pulse and temperature, and you'll be given an internal examination to see how far your cervix has dilated. She may record the fetal heart on an electronic monitor for up to 30 minutes.

• You'll be asked for a urine sample, which

will be tested for protein and sugar.
- You can then have a shower or bath if you like, and make yourself comfortable in the delivery room with the help of your birth partner and the midwife.

- If you have any questions or you want to discuss your birthplan (*see p.240*) and make your feelings known to the staff, now is the time to remind them of your preferences.

BREATHING FOR LABOUR AND BIRTH

If you have practised a relaxation technique (*see p.140*) and have learnt to recognize the different types or levels of breathing, now is the time to put them into practice. Your birth assistant will be able to help you by reminding you when your breathing is too rapid or your shoulders are tense. Your birth assistant can help by tapping out a rhythm or using words like "breathe, breathe, pant, pant, blow".

Early first stage
The contractions in the early stages will probably be gentle and you should be able to breathe deeply and evenly throughout. Greet each contraction with a slow, even breath out.

Late first stage
Take your opening breath out and then try to breathe above the contractions; light, short breaths that hardly seem to involve the lower parts of your body at all. Take a deep breath and relax when the contraction is over.

Transition
If you want to push too early, try panting – but without hyperventilating and starving your body of oxygen. Breathe through your mouth. If you are dizzy, your partner can cup his hands over your nose and mouth while you breathe.

Second stage
This requires the most natural breathing pattern. Take a deep breath and hold it while bearing down; let your pelvic floor bulge outwards. The push should be long and smooth. Repeat if the contraction is still intense; relax when it ends.

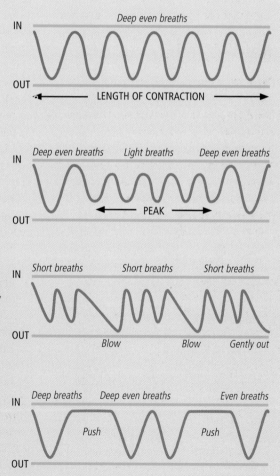

The first stage of labour

During this stage the cervix opens out (dilates) to allow the baby's head to pass through. Before it dilates, the cervix becomes thinned and softened and is gradually pulled up by the contracting uterine muscle. The muscle of the upper segment of the uterus contracts and puts pressure on to the lower segment, which in turn transmits the pull of the contractions to the cervix. As a result, once the cervix has stretched, it dilates with each contraction until the entire cervical canal is eliminated. You're then fully dilated.

The degrees of dilatation of the cervix have been standardized so that it can be described accurately and progress can be charted. If you ask the midwife how your labour is progressing, she'll probably respond in terms of the number of centimetres/inches your cervix has dilated or perhaps with the number of fingers (one finger is the equivalent of about 1cm (⅓in). Dilatation is normally given in one-centimetre increments up to 10cm (4in). When the cervix is said to be fully dilated it is approximately 10cm (4in) in diameter. This is the completion of the first stage of labour, though in real terms the first stage often moves gradually and smoothly into the second stage without punctuation.

BACKACHE LABOUR

If your baby is in the posterior position, its head may be pressing against your sacrum. This usually results in a long, erratic labour accompanied by backache. In this position the baby's head is not properly flexed and a wider part presents. However, the baby usually rotates before passing through the birth canal and the birth itself is normal. If your backache is particularly bad, there are ways to relieve it.

- Keep moving, and during contractions take up a position in which the pressure is taken off your back, for example on all fours, leaning into a chair, or rocking backwards and forwards.
- Nullify the pressure with counterpressure. Your birth assistant can apply pressure with fists or something round such as a tennis ball against your back.

- Apply a hot-water bottle to the lower part of your back between contractions.
- Don't lie flat on your back; the baby's head then presses onto your spine.
- Ask your birth assistant to massage your buttocks and your lower back (*see p. 143*).

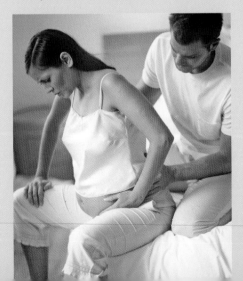

Relieving backache
Your partner can help to relieve the discomfort of backache by firmly massaging your lower back and sacrum area during labour.

Examinations during labour

If you've asked for an epidural, an anaesthetist will visit you after the admission procedure. If not, you'll be left with your partner or birth assistant and a midwife will be with you or available throughout your labour.

The fetal heart will be regularly monitored either by fetoscope, sonicaid or a machine (*see p.200*); you should be able to hear it too. You'll be given internal examinations about every four hours to check progress if all is going well. Examinations may be more frequent if there are problems or if the midwife is concerned. The midwife will do this while you are sitting up or lying on your side on the bed. Let her know which position you prefer. It is more difficult for the midwife to examine you while you're standing.

The midwife who examines you may or may not be one of the team who has been looking after you throughout. She will let you know that it is time to examine you and will tell you how things are going. Ask her, or get your partner to ask her, if you don't understand something. If you feel that your contractions are getting longer and stronger and you haven't had an internal examination for a while, then ask for one. It is quite cheering to find that your cervical dilatation has progressed between examinations. There's not usually any problem about your companion being allowed to stay with you while you have internal examinations, but it is your choice.

You may be asked questions during an internal examination or while you're having a contraction. Concentrate on what you are doing and answer afterwards.

WHAT HAPPENS TO YOUR CERVIX

During the first stage of labour, the cervix must be stretched thin and needs to open wide so your baby's head can pass through.

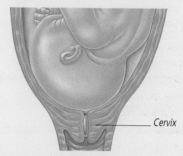

Latent phase
Your cervix remains about 2cm (¾in) long until contractions start thinning it out (effacing).

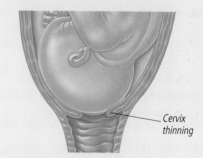

Active phase
When the cervical canal is thinned out, further contractions will widen (dilate) your cervix.

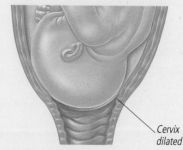

Transitional phase
The last part of your cervix at the front has opened to 10cm (4in). You are now fully dilated.

ADVICE TO BIRTH ASSISTANT FOR FIRST STAGE

- During pre-labour, encourage her to sleep and to conserve her strength when she can. You may see a burst of energy, which is the nesting instinct, but do tell her firmly to rest and put her feet up as much as possible.
- In the early stages of labour while the membranes haven't ruptured, encourage her to take a warm bath and help her to get in and out of the tub so that she doesn't slip. If the membranes have ruptured, a shower is best.
- Unless she is feeling nauseous, encourage her to eat and drink as she wants. Natural fruit juice and honey contain sugars that will give her plenty of energy. You should try to have something to eat too, as there may not be time later.
- When the contractions begin you should time them for her and note the interval between them (from the end of one to the beginning of another) and how long each contraction lasts. Put your hand on her abdomen so that you can feel the peak of the contraction.
- One of your most important roles is to coach her through the contractions, giving comfort and support. Never criticize; use positive words and praise as much as you can. Don't be offended if she turns away from you and seeks reassurance from the midwife. She is seeking help from the professional and not rejecting you.
- She will find it very soothing if you wipe her face. Your touch is comforting – try massaging her back or her abdomen gently, or just hold her hand.
- Be watchful for any signs of tension in her neck, shoulders and forehead, encourage her to relax and remind her how to do it. She should keep her mouth loose between contractions, so if you see any signs of tension ask her to close her mouth and drop her jaw.
- If she is up and mobile, remind her to empty her bladder every hour. If she gets up and moves about,

stay near her because any kind of activity can increase the contractions. Go with her when she goes to the toilet, and stay with her in the cubicle if she does not mind or wait by the door.

- Observe her moods and fit in with them. If she wants to stay quiet, then do so, but if she wants to be distracted, play a game of cards or Scrabble.
- When you arrive at the hospital and she is having contractions, go directly to the labour ward. The important thing is to move her as little as possible and get her settled as comfortably and as quickly as you can. Try to prevent anything that makes her anxious or interrupts her control of the labour.
- You'll be able to stay with your partner during the admissions procedure, but if things are still in the very early stages, this might be a good time to slip out for a bite to eat. Your partner is going to need you with her all the time later on.
- If the medical staff suggest painkilling drugs, make sure that she knows what is being offered and what they are for. If she feels like trying to hang on, help her do so, but always remember that there is absolutely no reason why she should not be given drugs if they are medically indicated in her case. If she asks for pain relief, don't discourage her unduly – remember that she is the one in labour, and it is her decision.
- If you're at home, the midwife will probably be on her own for most of the time, so be ready to assist whenever she asks. Do as she says as quickly and calmly as possible.
- When labour is well established, you could place your hand on her abdomen so that you can feel it begin to tighten and know when the next contraction is coming. As the uterus starts to harden and rise, tell her to take a deep breath. You can make sure that she is not caught off-guard by contractions and therefore she will be able to control them better.

POSITIONS FOR THE FIRST STAGE

There is no single "correct" position for labour; experiment and find the most comfortable position for you. Move around and keep trying new positions, using the furniture or your partner for support if you like. Many women like to move around and when the contraction starts, take up their chosen position.

Staying upright
This encourages contractions during the first stage. You will feel more comfortable if your knees are slightly apart and your back is straight. Use a cushion over the back of a chair to lean against.

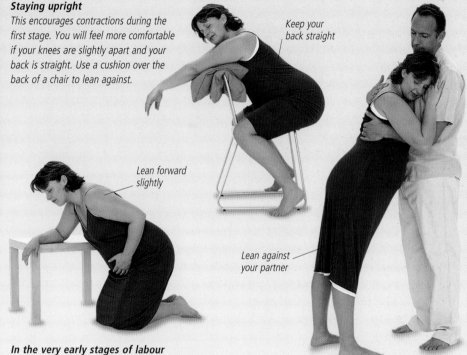

Keep your back straight

Lean forward slightly

Lean against your partner

In the very early stages of labour
Stop what you are doing during the contraction and support yourself on whatever is close by. If the surface is high, kneel down and lean slightly forwards.

Using your partner
Lean onto your birth assistant. The weight of the baby will be taken off your spine and the contractions will be most efficient in this upright position. He can massage your back.

Don't arch your back

If you have backache
Kneel on all fours and rock backwards and forwards during contractions. Don't arch your back. Lean forwards between contractions onto your folded arms or sit back on your haunches.

The transitional stage

This is the period from the end of the first stage of labour to the beginning of the second stage. Not all women experience it as a well defined, distinct stage of labour, but some do and it is better to be prepared. It rarely lasts for more than an hour, often much less, but it can be quite hard to cope with.

Coming at the end of several hours in the first stage, some women become discouraged and feel that they can't go on without pain relief. There may be some shaking and shivering, which is normal and physiological. Simply because of all the hormonal changes that are going on you may feel some irritability and ill-temper, which is also absolutely normal. Some women become so nauseous that they want to vomit. If this happens to you don't resist this urge because you will feel a lot better afterwards.

You may feel excited and restless; every position seems uncomfortable. You may feel anxious for your own safety and for your baby's, and you may feel sleepy between contractions because most of the oxygen in your body is being taken up by the uterus and the baby, and your brain is relatively short of it.

Breathing techniques

Some women feel the urge to push during this transitional stage but don't bear down until your midwife has confirmed that your cervix is fully dilated (see p.174). If you feel a strong urge to push but your midwife says it is too soon to do so, use the panting and blowing breathing technique (see p.142) until the midwife tells you it is safe to start to push.

For most women the end of the transition stage is marked by a noticeable change in the pattern of breathing. You may grunt involuntarily, and this is because you will start to feel the urge to bear down. The need to push becomes very strong. Do ask your birth assistant to alert the staff and tell them that you are ready to push. The midwife will confirm that your cervix has dilated 10cm (4in) and that the second stage is beginning. Your baby is about to be born.

ADVICE TO BIRTH ASSISTANT

- Try to get her to relax. Refrain from asking questions and remove perspiration if she's sweating a lot.
- If she tells you not to touch her, refrain but stay near the bed. If she feels sick and wants to vomit, get a basin and encourage her to do so. Always praise her.
- If her legs start to tremble, put her socks on her and hold her legs firmly.
- If you notice that she is beginning to grunt and make pushing movements, let the midwife know immediately. This is a difficult time for your partner, and you can encourage her by explaining that you think she is in transition, stage two is beginning and the baby will soon be born.
- You will know that the delivery is imminent when the midwife says that the head is crowning – it is beginning to emerge from the vaginal opening.

POSITIONS DURING THE TRANSITION

Transition is a difficult stage in which to find a comfortable position. Contractions seem relentless but if you understand that your baby will be born soon, that should give you the encouragement and confidence to stay calm and patient. You probably won't feel like moving around so much but try to change positions every now and again. Your birth assistant can help by suggesting positions.

Using your birth assistant
Leaning forwards onto your partner can make you feel more secure. Put your feet on a stool or chair, and keep your knees wide apart.

Rest your head on your arms

Lean forwards

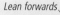

If the cervix is not fully dilated
If you feel the need to bear down, use gravity to slow the baby down while the cervix continues to dilate. Kneel down and either sit back on your haunches and rest your head in your arms against a low chair, or lean forward and put your head on your arms on the floor and your bottom in the air. This takes pressure off your lower back.

If you want to rest
Lie down on your side with cushions under your head and upper thigh. Keep your legs as wide apart as possible.

Keep legs apart

The second stage of labour

For a first baby the second stage generally doesn't last longer than two hours and it may be as little as five minutes. Bearing down is a reflex, an instinctive urge to push down, which is caused by the baby's head pressing on the pelvic floor and the rectum. You will know automatically to take a deep breath, so lowering your diaphragm, which exerts pressure on the uterus, will help the pushing. You then hold your breath, slightly bend your knees and strain downwards. Pushing is much harder if you are lying on your back. It is easier if you are upright, squatting, sitting up supported, on all fours, or on your knees, leaning against a chair or your partner. This way you have the force of gravity to help you. Your pushing should be smooth and continuous. All of the muscular effort should be down and out. It should be fairly slow and gradual so that the vaginal tissues and muscles are given time to stretch and accommodate your baby's head without tearing or making an episiotomy necessary. Even so, you can still tear.

Push during a contraction. Your pushing only helps the uterus to expel the baby. The involuntary muscles of the uterus can expel the baby on their own. So you help most by beginning your pushing effort with the peak intensity of each contraction. During pushing, the pelvic floor and the anal area should be as relaxed as possible, so try to relax this part of your body (*see p.122*). When you've finished a push you'll find two slow, deep breaths helpful, but don't relax too quickly at the end of a contraction as the baby will maintain its forward progress if you relax slowly.

ADVICE TO BIRTH ASSISTANT FOR SECOND STAGE

- Remind her to relax her pelvic floor during pushing. She should take two or three deep breaths and then push her hardest at the peak of contractions. Remind her that she should push in a strong, steady way.
- Remind her to look in the mirror so that she can see the baby emerging.
- If you are in hospital and are asked to leave the delivery room suddenly, do so without question. There may be a medical emergency and staff will have to move very fast. You cannot guarantee that you will not be in the way. Leave the delivery room but stay close by outside.
- Remind her to lie back and relax fully between contractions so that she conserves her strength for pushing.

- You are now more of an observer once the baby's head has crowned. The midwife will be the one who needs to coach your partner through the pushing stage.
- Don't expect your partner to communicate with you during the birth. She will be preoccupied and may not notice you for some time.
- When the baby is placed on your partner's stomach, if possible put your arms around them both to keep them warm and show her that you're still there.
- Be ready for your own and your partner's reactions. There may be tears, silence, whoops of joy, perhaps even squeamishness. It's all perfectly normal and understandable so don't feel you have to hold back your emotions.

POSITIONS FOR THE DELIVERY

You will know by now from your experience of labour so far what position is going to be most comfortable to give birth in. Take advice from your medical attendants; they will lead you through the pushing stage. Enjoy yourself and take your time. Your baby will soon be born.

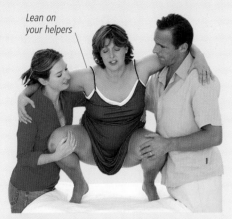

Lean on your helpers

Supported squat
Your partner can support you by taking your weight on his arms. He should keep his back straight, and his knees slightly bent.

Let your partner take your weight

Squatting
This opens up the pelvis, relaxes the pelvic floor and vaginal opening and uses the force of gravity to deliver the baby. To squat on a bed, you will need two helpers to support you so that you feel safe.

A common delivery position
Sit propped up with cushions, hold onto your knees and drop your chin on your chest. You can lie back and relax between each contraction and conserve your energy. You will be able to see the baby emerge.

Drop your chin

Lean back

Semi-upright position
If you feel happier being close to your partner during the delivery, you can lean back against him. His closeness will give you confidence and he can encourage you to push during contractions.

Birth is imminent

The first sign that your baby is soon to arrive is the bulging of your anus and perineum, caused by the pressure of the baby's head. With each contraction more and more of the baby's head appears at your vaginal opening, until it doesn't slip back at all between contractions. This is known as crowning. After crowning, the baby's head will be delivered in the next contraction or two.

It's normal to feel a stinging or burning sensation as the baby stretches the outlet of the birth canal. As soon as you feel it, stop bearing down, pant and allow the uterus to push the baby out on its own. This may be difficult as you'll probably still feel like pushing, but if you continue to push you run a greater risk of tearing or needing an episiotomy.

As you stop pushing, try to go limp. Make a conscious effort to relax the muscles of the perineal floor (*see p.122*). The burning or stinging sensation lasts for a short time and is immediately followed by a numb feeling as the baby's head stretches the vaginal tissues so thinly that the nerves are blocked, giving a natural anaesthetic effect. If the medical staff feel you are going to tear badly, this is the moment they may do an episiotomy (*see p.196*). As the baby's head is delivered, you will feel a sensation like toothpaste coming out of a tube. As soon as the head has emerged, the midwife will check that the umbilical cord is not around the baby's neck (*see p.186*).

When the head is delivered, the baby's back will be uppermost; his face is pointing towards your rectum. Almost immediately, however, he will start to rotate his

shoulders so that he is facing your right or left thigh. The direction depends on his position in the uterus. The midwife will wipe his eyes, nose and mouth with clean gauze, and remove any fluid from the nose and upper air passages.

Now there may be a breathing space when the uterine contractions stop for a few minutes. When they restart, you hardly need to push because within the next one or two contractions, your baby's shoulders will be born, followed by his body. Sometimes head and body are born in the one contraction.

Occasionally the baby's shoulders don't come out easily. The midwife will call for urgent help and an episiotomy may be needed. The midwife usually assists this last part of delivery by putting her thumbs and fingers under the armpits of your baby. She'll then lift him upwards towards your

YOUR BABY'S BIRTH

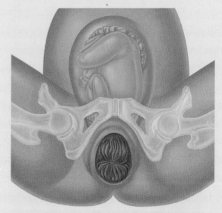

1 *As the baby's head crowns, the stinging sensation is followed by numbness as the vaginal tissues are stretched so thin that the nerves are blocked. The head then slips out.*

abdomen, holding him firmly as he will be slippery with blood and amniotic fluid. If you're feeling alert and you're in a position to do so, you can bend down and pull your baby out yourself and onto your abdomen.

Your baby may cry when first delivered and will be crying lustily a few seconds after birth. If the breathing is normal, there's absolutely no reason why you should not hold your baby immediately. Ask if you can lay the baby on your abdomen and keep him warm with your arms and those of your partner. If there's a danger of the baby being cold, all three of you can be kept warm with a blanket.

Your baby's birth
Once your baby's head is out, the midwife will gently guide him so that his shoulders can be delivered one at a time. The rest of your baby's body will then slide out. The pushing contractions stop and you'll feel a wonderful sense of release.

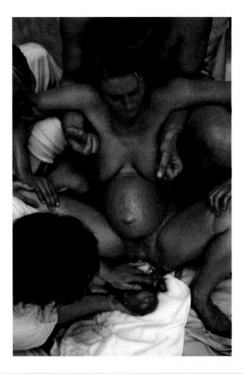

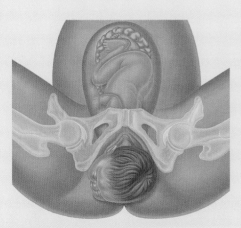

2 *The baby's head is born facing downwards towards the rectum, but the baby immediately turns to face your thigh to get into a good position for the birth of the body.*

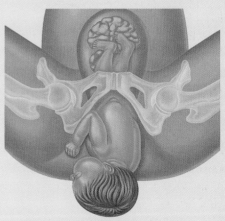

3 *The midwife will clear any fluid and mucus from the baby's air passages. The next uterine contraction is usually sufficient to deliver the shoulders and then the body.*

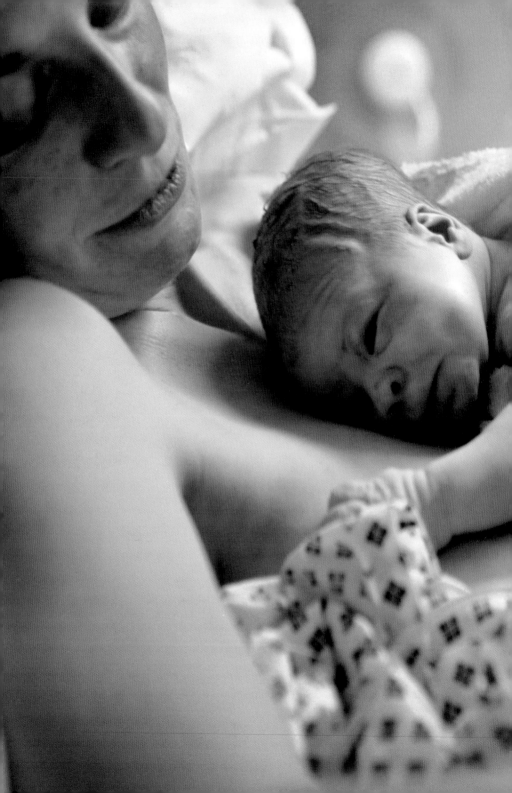

Your gentle stroking movements, your soothing voice and the sound of your heartbeat are all just what your baby needs at this moment. He may start to suckle spontaneously.

Your baby will probably be a bluish colour at first and may be covered with the white greasy vernix (see p.85). He will have streaks of blood on his head and body and, depending on your delivery, his head may be elongated after the journey down the birth canal. The midwife will make a check of his general condition (see p.214). If there is fluid in the mouth or nose or air passages, the midwife will want to make sure that it's cleared and breathing is normal. She will suck it out. If the baby doesn't start to breathe immediately, the midwife will take him and give him oxygen. Don't be alarmed at the sudden activity. As soon as your baby's breathing is normal, he will be returned to you to hold.

The third stage of labour

When the baby is born the uterus rests and after about 15 minutes starts to contract again, comparatively painlessly, to expel the placenta. This is the third stage of labour. When the baby's shoulder appears the midwife usually gives the mother an injection in the thigh of syntometrine, a synthetic hormone that increases the contractions of the uterus to prevent major haemorrhage. Oxytocin, produced naturally in response to seeing and touching your baby, but most of all to putting him to the breast, does the same job. The injection is usually administered in a hospital delivery, although the midwife or doctor will ask your permission first.

In the third stage of labour the placenta detaches itself from the uterine wall. The large blood vessels, about the thickness of a pencil, that run to and from the placenta are simply torn across. Most women do not bleed because the muscle fibres of the uterus are arranged in a criss-cross fashion. When the uterus contracts down, these muscles tighten around the blood vessels, preventing them from bleeding. This is why it is absolutely essential that the uterus contracts

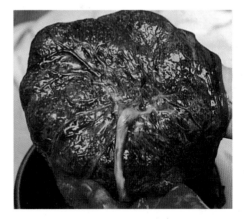

Your first moments together
You've waited so long for this – the moment when you can hold your baby for the first time and give her a cuddle. Your midwife will probably lay the baby on your tummy or give her to you to hold while the cord is being clamped and cut.

Delivery of the placenta
One or two pushes should expel the placenta. The midwife will put one hand on your uterus and will gently pull on the cord to ease the placenta out.

down into a hard ball once the placenta has been expelled. The uterus can be kept tightly contracted by massaging it for an hour or so after the third stage is complete.

When the placenta is delivered

The placenta slips out with a gentle squelch. It looks rather like a piece of liver and many women like to look at it and examine it. It is an amazing organ – it has been the life-support system for your baby for nine months. Once the placenta is delivered, the midwife will examine it to make sure it's complete. If any of the placenta has been retained it can be a cause of haemorrhage later on (see p.210) and may need to be surgically removed.

You may shiver profoundly after delivery of the placenta. After delivery of my second child I was shivering so much and my teeth were chattering so that I couldn't speak and couldn't breathe properly. My explanation for this reaction is that for nine months I had a little furnace inside me, producing a lot of heat, and my body had adjusted to take account of that heat production by turning my own thermostat down slightly. When my baby left my body, I was deprived of that heat and I started shivering to raise my body temperature. The shivering usually passes in about half an hour, during which time the body temperature has been brought back up to normal and your own thermostat reset. Often the muscles in your legs feel quite sore for a day or two.

Clamping the cord

There is no need for the unseemly rush to clamp the cord that there used to be 30 years ago when I first qualified. The cord will only need to be clamped and cut at once if it is looped tightly around the baby's neck. This is quite common, and the baby will then be delivered very quickly. Usually the midwife is able to slip the cord out from around the baby's head and the delivery can proceed without immediate clamping. It's generally believed that the baby benefits from the return of placental blood through the umbilical cord and that it should not be clamped until it stops pulsating. (Blood can flow from the placenta to the baby only if the baby is at a lower level than the uterus.) When the time is right, the cord is divided between a pair of clamps placed 13–15cm (5–6in) from the baby's navel.

Put your baby to the breast

Now the three of you should be left alone. Put your baby to the breast as soon as possible – preferably in the first five minutes and even before the cord is clamped if that's an option. Breast-feeding releases oxytocin, which helps the uterus to contract, and the colostrum in your breasts (see p.221) contains antibodies that will guard against some forms of gastric infection. Don't worry if he doesn't want to suckle yet, just concentrate on getting to know him.

A newborn is usually alert during the first hour after a normal birth, and will look intently at you if you hold him 20–25cm (8–10in) from your face. He can focus at this distance, which is the distance between your face and his when you

Holding your baby
While the placenta is being expelled, you can hold your baby for the first time.

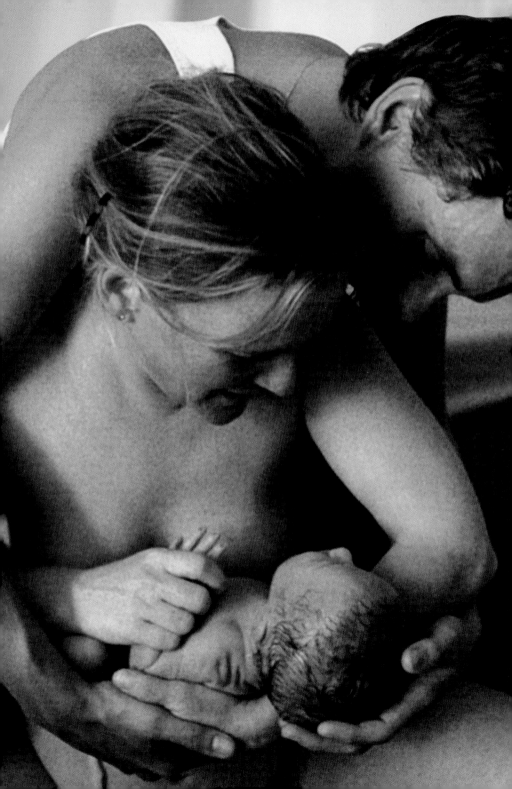

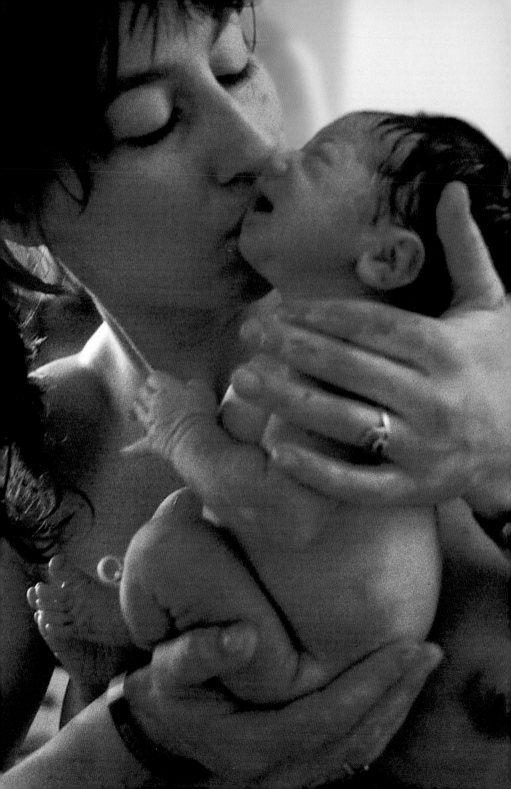

cradle him to the breast. Presently you will be washed, stitched if necessary and asked to pass urine to check that everything is working all right. The midwives will wipe your baby, weigh him and put him in the crib ready to take to the postnatal ward.

Sudden delivery

If you are alone, or if your doctor or midwife has not arrived when the baby is about to be born, try to pant or blow until they arrive. You should be able to keep this up for five minutes even though the urge to push plus the pressure from the baby's head crowning may make it difficult. Whatever you do, don't try to hold your legs together to delay the birth, and don't allow anyone else to do this; it could harm your baby. If your baby is coming and you cannot delay it, don't try to interfere. If you are totally alone, sitting on the floor in a semi-upright position is probably the safest and most comfortable one for you to be in. Holding onto something firm with your arms is both sensible and efficient. Make sure that your baby is delivered onto something soft and clean (a sheet, large towel or tablecloth would do). If you can manage, you may even help the baby out yourself once the head has been delivered and the shoulders are clear of the vagina. After that sit or lie down with your baby's skin close to your own; your body heat will keep the baby warm. Cover yourselves with a sheet or blanket and put the baby to suckle at your breast while you wait for help to arrive.

Your baby is born
You'll never forget this first moment. You'll feel lost in wonder at this little human being, complete with perfect features and tiny hands and feet.

Neonatal unit

If there is a problem with the baby, such as low birthweight, he may be taken to the neonatal unit (NNU) for special care. You may feel disappointed that you can't touch and feed him but the staff will be sympathetic, so ask to be allowed to help with the care of your baby. Ask questions of the staff and expect answers that help you to understand what is happening. If you find you can't communicate effectively, ask your partner or a friend to talk to the paediatrician, or sister in charge. You will be encouraged to breast-feed your baby if you want to, even though he is in an incubator. The hospital will supply you with a pump to express your milk for him and it will be fed to him by tube. Touch him as much as you can so that you gain confidence in handling your tiny baby.

When it is twins

Labour is no more painful with a twin delivery than with a single baby. Almost certainly you will be advised to have the babies in hospital in case you need extra help with the birth, or if the babies are not presenting properly (*see p.157*). There is no reason why your partner shouldn't stay with you during the delivery, and you should discuss this with your midwife during the last trimester. Your consultant will probably recommend an epidural (*see p.193*) in case the second twin needs help and to reduce the chances of needing an emergency general anaesthetic.

There is only one first stage of labour if you're having twins. Once the cervix is fully dilated and you're able to push, both babies are pushed out, one after the other. There are two second stages, although the second one will be short, especially if the second baby is smaller. Most second babies are born ten to 30 minutes after the first.

Emotionally a twin birth is different from a single birth. You'll hardly appreciate the delivery of the second baby, such is the feeling of triumph and joy when the first baby is born. Once the first baby is born, the midwife will examine you to see how the second baby is lying. The contractions will begin again after a few minutes and the membranes will be artificially ruptured. After the second baby is delivered you will be given an injection of syntometrine in your thigh to ensure that the uterus contracts properly and to speed up the third stage – the birth of the placenta.

Feeding your new twins
Breast-feeding your twins together is good for them and you. Your breasts produce more highly nutritious milk when your babies suckle at the same time.

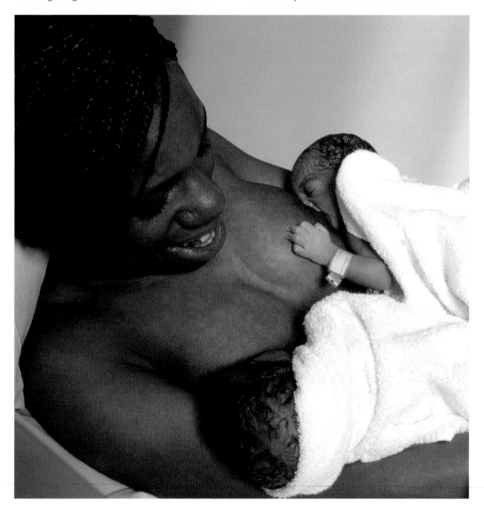

Pain relief in labour

For many women, particularly first-time mothers, excitement about their baby's birth may be overshadowed by worry about pain during labour.

The pain of labour

The experience is different for everyone, but the amount of pain actually felt almost always has a strong relationship with what is expected. Of course you should be realistic, but your expectations can be greatly modified by what you learn, the information you are given, and how confident you feel when you go into labour. This is why antenatal classes and breathing exercises, which give you the knowledge that you have some control over your body and pain, are so important.

Everyone agrees that fear and ignorance cause tension, stress and anxiety, all of which make pain worse, and may even create pain where there is very little. Information, knowledge and support can go a long way to dispel fear and anxiety, and will also help to ease pain. There's no question that pain can be relieved with drugs, but to my mind the best forms of pain relief are information, a calm state of mind and moral support. Armed with these you will find that the pain you feel is less, and that you may be strong enough to cope without resorting to analgesics or anaesthetics, which might dim your awareness of what's going on.

Doctors and midwives believe that an important part of their job is to make labour as pain-free as possible and if they feel you are in difficulty they will be keen to offer you a range of analgesics. However, they will not force anything on you. It is a good idea to discuss pain relief at the antenatal clinic early in your pregnancy, to make your preferences clear (*see p.72*) and have them recorded in your notes and birth plan (*see p.240*). Always remember to state alternatives in case things don't go according to plan.

Of course it's impossible to know your own pain threshold in advance and not every problem can be predicted. So it is important to go into labour with an open mind and to accept the pain relief offered if it is considered essential. Whatever happens, don't feel guilty; not everyone has a trouble-free labour and birth. Your labour isn't a test, and the use of drugs may even be essential for you to be able deliver your baby.

Decision to accept pain relief

There are two important considerations about the use of painkilling drugs in labour. With most drugs, whether they're sedatives that make you feel calm and sleepy, hypnotics, which actually send you to sleep, or narcotics that make you feel light-headed and cut off from the normal world, you will lose some awareness of what is happening around you. Many women want to experience every second of giving birth and any interference with their level of awareness is unacceptable. The second important factor is that most drugs will cross the placenta to the baby and will be in a higher concentration in the baby's blood than in the mother's blood.

Many mothers find this unacceptable. Bearing both of these things in mind, and after getting as much information as you need, make up your mind about your attitude to having pain-killing drugs in your labour.

A useful tip is to wait a little before accepting drugs. Some good news and moral support may be enough to get you over a sticky patch. Ask how far dilated you are. If you feel you are making good progress and can hang on, that may increase your resolve. Some encouraging words from your partner will give you added strength. So give yourself about 15 minutes after you feel you may want some pain relief before actually having it.

During that time you may make quite good progress. You might even have got through the most painful parts of labour and have only a little way to go. You may be astonished at your own strength and resilience and feel that you can manage perfectly well without drugs.

Anaesthetics

A general anaesthetic is never used during a normal birth, but a local or regional anaesthetic may be given to dull your

Using Entonox
Used properly, Entonox, often known as gas and air, gives a mild level of pain relief. You can take Entonox via a mouthpiece, as below, or a face mask.

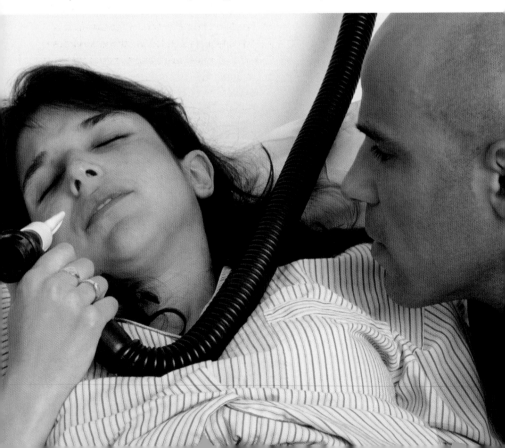

ANALGESICS IN LABOUR

Type of drug	Action	Effect on mother and/or baby
Narcotics (morphine, pethidine)	Sedate and relieve anxiety. Possibly relieve pain during the first stage of labour.	Reduce consciousness and tend to make the labour longer. Crosses the placenta in five minutes and can depress respiration at birth. Sucking may be inefficient (*see p.215*). Can produce nausea in the mother.
Inhalation analgesia (Entonox)	Relieves pain. Can cause drowsiness if allowed to accumulate.	Depresses alertness but this returns once the effects have worn off. Makes you light-headed while breathing in the gas. No significant effect on the baby.

conscious appreciation of pain. Anaesthetic is injected into a nerve root to numb the part of the body that the nerve supplies. The most widely used local anaesthetic is the epidural (*see p.194*). There is also the pudendal block, a local anaesthetic injection that numbs the lower part of the vagina before forceps or ventouse deliveries. A needle is guided through the vagina to make an injection round the pudendal nerve.

Analgesics

These are drugs that relieve pain. They work by numbing the pain centre of the brain. Inhalation analgesia (sometimes erroneously known as gas and air) is in fact a mixture of nitrous oxide and oxygen called Entonox. It is self-administered and you can inhale it half a minute before the peak of a contraction. You may become light-headed while inhaling it, but regain full consciousness a few seconds later. You will be given the opportunity to practise with the machine in your antenatal classes. Even if you don't use it successfully during labour, it gives you something to concentrate on while you are having contractions, which can be helpful.

Pethidine is a narcotic given by injection in varying dosages during the first stage. It takes about 20 minutes to work and is sometimes combined with other drugs. Pethidine relaxes you and relieves your anxiety, but its painkilling effect is variable. The safest time to administer the drug is six to eight hours before delivery. As this is difficult to calculate and the drug wears off in about two hours, it is probably best for those women who are nervous and anxious during the early first stage of labour.

Epidural anaesthesia

The epidural (see overleaf) prevents pain being felt in the abdominal area by acting as a "nerve block" in the spine, removing all sensation from your waist to your knees. It probably has no effect on the fetus directly, but it may have an affect on the length of your labour.

One of the reasons why the epidural has become so popular is that it fulfils all the criteria of a good pain reliever but it does not interfere with your awareness or consciousness in any way. There are very few side effects associated with the majority of epidural anaesthetics, and for many women it is a perfect answer.

Hypnobirthing

If you choose hypnosis for pain relief during labour you'll need to be prepared by a trained hypnotherapist during five or so 30-minute visits throughout pregnancy. Hypnosis is a natural and safe state of profound relaxation. You remain fully present and aware during the birth. Research shows that hypnosis can lessen the pain of labour, shorten its length and reduce incidence of postnatal depression.

TENS

This stands for Transcutaneous Nerve Stimulation and is a means of relieving labour pain by stimulating production of the body's natural painkillers – endorphins

– and by blocking pain sensation with an electric current. The electrodes are placed on the woman's body and she is able to regulate the intensity of the current herself. TENS has been used successfully, but it does not help everyone, in particular not those women who experience lots of pain. TENS doesn't relieve all of the pain but what remains is possibly easier to bear. A try-out before labour is advisable to make sure you know how to operate it properly.

Acupuncture

I would recommend acupuncture for pain relief only if you have successfully used it in the past. The acupuncturist must be practised at giving pain relief in labour.

HAVING AN EPIDURAL

An epidural takes about ten to 20 minutes for a skilled anaesthetist to set up. The analgesic effect is usually felt in just a few minutes and lasts for about two hours but can be "topped up" when necessary.

Setting up an epidural
You'll be asked to empty your bladder, then to lie down on your left side and pull your legs up to make as tight a ball as you can. Your lower back

will be washed with cold spirit and you'll have an injection of local anaesthetic. A small hole is made in your back with a solid needle and a hollow needle is then inserted in its place. Once the epidural space is located, a fine catheter is threaded through the hollow needle and into the epidural space, leaving a length of catheter protruding from your back. The catheter is secured to your skin along its length with paper tape. The local anaesthetic is then given by syringe down the catheter and the opening is sealed.

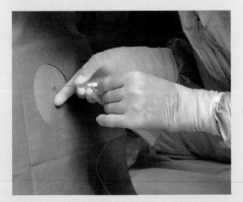
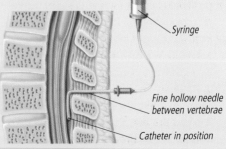

Syringe

Fine hollow needle between vertebrae

Catheter in position

ADMINISTERING THE EPIDURAL

Medical intervention

Hospital childbirth has been revolutionized by procedures that have been widely adopted as routine practice. All offer advantages; a few carry small risks. None of them should be used unless there are good medical reasons. Most people believe that the convenience of the staff or even of the mother should not be the sole justification for using these procedures.

Episiotomy

In an episiotomy, which takes place during the second stage of labour, an incision is made in the perineum between the vaginal opening and the anus to facilitate delivery of the baby. It is the most common operation in the western world.

The cut is made with scissors under a local anaesthetic just as the baby's head appears. If it is done too early, before the perineum has thinned out, muscles, skin and blood vessels are damaged and the bleeding may be profuse. Also the tissues are crushed by the scissors as they are cut. This leads to bruising, swelling and slow healing and accounts for a great deal of the pain and discomfort that often follows episiotomy. There is also the possibility that

ADVANTAGES AND DISADVANTAGES OF AN EPIDURAL

Advantages

- An epidural provides complete pain relief without dulling any of your mental faculties.
- It has a tendency to slow down labour, which can be useful.
- No other local anaesthetic will be necessary should you need forceps, vacuum extraction or episiotomy at the last minute.
- It allows you to participate in your birth if you have a Caesarean, and the baby needs less resuscitation than with a general anaesthetic.
- As it lowers blood pressure it is ideal for women with pre-eclampsia or high blood pressure.
- It can be topped up with extra anaesthetic or allowed to wear off near the delivery so that you can control the actual birth. The contractions at this stage may be a bit of a shock, though, if you haven't experienced any until then.
- It reduces the amount of work done by the lungs in labour and so can benefit women who suffer from any form of heart or lung disease.

Disadvantages

- The lowering of blood pressure may make you feel dizzy and nauseous. This is more likely if you lie on your back so turn onto your side.
- There is the possibility of a post-anaesthetic headache that lasts a few hours after delivery.
- There is a possibility of an episiotomy and a forceps delivery. Depending on the concentration of the anaesthetic, there may be a loss of muscle power and of the sensation of the contractions. This results in a slower second stage because you will be entirely dependent on the instructions of the midwife as to when to push the baby out. The length of the second stage is the factor that determines whether or not forceps are used.
- If the mother's blood pressure drops, the amount of blood supplying the placenta is reduced and so the oxygen supply to the baby is lowered.
- If an epidural is allowed to wear off near delivery, the contractions may come as a nasty shock.
- Not all epidurals are effective.

EXPERIENCE OF EPISIOTOMY

Sheila Kitzinger, in her study of 2,000 women who had episiotomies, came to the following conclusions about the procedure:

• Episiotomies were more painful than a tear.
• Women found it more difficult to get into a comfortable position to hold the baby after an episiotomy.
• The pain distracted them during breast-feeding.
• An episiotomy was more likely to give pain or discomfort during sexual intercourse even three months after delivery.
• Two-thirds of the women had never discussed episiotomy with medical staff during pregnancy. Some had tried but had been unsuccessful.
• About half the episiotomies had been done when the perineum was not sufficiently thinned out.
• More than half the women had not been instructed to release the vagina and pelvic floor muscles, but had been encouraged to push instead, which made the episiotomy more necessary.
• About one-quarter of the women had not been told to stop pushing while the head was being born to give the vagina a chance to thin out.
• More than one-third of the women were never given a reason for the episiotomy.
• Some women found the stitching painful but when they complained they were told (incorrectly) that there were no nerve endings in that part of the body.

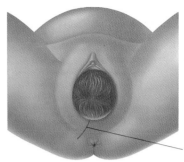
— *Medio-lateral*

Episiotomy incision
The incision is generally made from the back of the vagina and then down and outward. This is called a medio-lateral incision.

the integrity of the pelvic floor can be damaged if the muscle fibres are not correctly aligned.

If the vagina and perineum are stitched too tightly a woman may experience discomfort when intercourse is resumed. You might like to have it recorded in your notes that you wish to avoid having an episiotomy if it is at all possible and you can add it to your birthplan.

If medical staff indicate that they think an episiotomy is necessary during labour, you or your birth partner should ask why it's being done.

Avoiding an episiotomy

One of the best ways to avoid the necessity for an episiotomy is to deliver your baby in as upright a position as you possibly can (*see p.181*). Tell your midwife early in labour that you want to find a good position for the second stage of labour and in particular that you'd like to avoid lying on your back. Together with your birth partner, your midwife will then be ready to help give you the support you need when the time comes.

If you learn how to relax the muscles of the pelvic floor antenatally and allow your vaginal tissues and perineum to bulge out (see p.122) you can probably avoid a tear. Familiarity with the sensation when the baby's head bulges or "crowns" will mean that you will realize that you are starting to tighten up in the second stage and you can try to do something about it.

Having an epidural anaesthetic may increase the possibility of having an episiotomy. If you do opt for an epidural, there is no reason why an episiotomy is automatically necessary, but you will need to make your views known to your midwife and your birth partner.

It is also a good idea to try to have the end of the second stage well under your control by relaxing the pelvic floor muscles and not pushing down too hard when the baby's head is delivered. I had an epidural twice, but on neither occasion did I have an episiotomy.

Induction

This is the artificial "starting off" of labour. Your labour will be induced should it fail to start on its own or if for some reason your doctor decides that you need to deliver the baby early. If you are in any doubt about why your doctor is suggesting induction, ask for a detailed explanation.

Induction is usually planned in advance; depending on the hospital, you may be admitted the night before or you may simply come into the hospital on the day. Induction is often introduced gradually, first with prostaglandin pessaries, then if necessary, by rupturing the membranes (ARM), and finally, if things are going too slowly, with an oxytocin drip.

REASONS FOR AN EPISIOTOMY

An episiotomy will be necessary if:
- The perineum hasn't had time to stretch slowly – breathing exercises and massage can help you with this.
- The baby's head is too large for the vaginal opening.
- You aren't able to control your pushing so that you can stop when necessary and then push gradually and smoothly. An episiotomy will deliver the baby quickly if you have difficulty with co-ordination and control of pushing in the second stage.
- The baby is distressed.
- You have a forceps or ventouse (vacuum extraction) delivery.
- Yours is a breech birth.

Prostaglandin pessaries

No one knows exactly how labour starts, but pessaries or a gel containing prostaglandins, which are made up of various hormones that have an effect on a pregnant woman's uterus, are used to induce labour.

The use of prostaglandin pessaries inserted into the vagina is the least invasive method of starting labour and leaves you free to move around. The pessaries can be inserted at any time of day, although most units put them in at night, and they usually take full effect after about six hours. Sometimes a single pesssary may be enough, but more than one may be needed to get things going. In 50 per cent of cases the prostaglandin pessaries may be supplemented with rupturing the membranes (ARM) and an oxytocin drip.

Rupture of the membranes

Also known as ARM or amniotomy, rupturing the membranes is only done if the cervix is sufficiently open and the head is low in the pelvis. It doesn't in itself stimulate contractions although they may start spontaneously. However, ARM often needs supplementing with oxytocin to stimulate contractions, because labour must begin within 24 hours to avoid the risk of infection.

An instrument that looks not unlike a crochet hook is inserted into the neck of the womb and a small opening is made in the membrane so that the waters escape. For most women this is a painless procedure. Labour usually reaches full intensity quickly after ARM because the baby's head is no longer cushioned and it presses hard against the cervix, which encourages the uterus to contract.

Amniotomy was until fairly recently almost a routine procedure during the preparation for any labour. If left alone, the waters may rupture spontaneously at any stage of labour. There are two major disadvantages of amniotomy. The first is that it makes the labour proceed more intensely than it would normally. Also, if the baby has the cord around its neck, the loss of fluid increases pressure and can affect the flow of blood through the cord to the baby.

Besides being a method of induction, amniotomy will be performed if an electrode is to be attached to the baby's head to monitor its heartbeat *(see p.200)*; if the baby's heart rate goes down, the amniotic fluid can be examined for traces of meconium, the first bowel movements of the baby. Meconium in the fluid can indicate fetal distress.

Oxytocin-induced labour

The hormone oxytocin, which is produced by the pituitary gland in the brain, stimulates the uterus to start contracting. It is therefore given in a synthetic form to start labour off and to keep it going.

Oxytocin is normally given via a drip inserted into a vein. Ask for it to be inserted in the arm you use least and check that you have a long tube connecting you to the drip. You should then have more

RUPTURE OF MEMBRANES

The bag of waters usually ruptures naturally towards the end of the first stage of labour. Before it breaks, it provides a cushion for the baby's head as it presses against the cervix (right). Once the membranes have ruptured (far right), the contractions increase in intensity because the baby's head is now resting hard against the cervix. This speeds up labour, which is why amniotomy may be performed if progress is slow.

Amniotic fluid cushions the baby's head

After an amniotomy the head presses on the cervix

room to move around, even if just on the bed. The drip can be turned down if you go into strong labour quickly and the cervix becomes half dilated. The drip won't be removed from your arm until after the baby is born as the uterus needs to keep contracting to expel the placenta and then prevent bleeding *(see p.185)*.

The contractions you experience while on an oxytocin drip are often stronger, longer and more painful, with shorter periods of relaxation in between them. Unfortunately this may mean the need for painkilling drugs is greater. Also, the blood supply to the uterus is temporarily shut off during each strong contraction, which may be detrimental to the baby.

Reasons for induction

When induction was first available it was frequently used for hospital or social convenience. Induction was sometimes planned to suit working hours or changes in shifts, for example. In the sixties and seventies, obstetrics went through a phase of over-zealous high-tech intervention, when there was a great vogue for induced labours, especially in older mothers who, at that time, were much less common than they are today. Oxytocin-induced labour was once used in as many as 40–50 per cent of deliveries.

Given that the rate of success with this form of induction is only about 85 per cent, its routine use cannot be justified, and most modern obstetricians believe that less than a few per cent of pregnant women require it. Nowadays fewer than one in five labours is induced by any method and I'd like to reassure you that induction is fine for you and your baby,

provided it's done strictly for medical reasons, such as pre-eclampsia. If properly handled it needn't be more painful or difficult than natural labour. If it does become too painful, you can ask for an epidural or other pain relief.

Only five per cent of babies actually come on the due date and it's hard for some doctors and quite a lot of mothers to remain philosophical when that magic date passes. Both are concerned in case the baby is "postmature", or late. The fear is that the placenta may be becoming inadequate to support the baby and the baby is outgrowing its food supply.

Very few babies are truly overdue, however; 80 per cent of all babies who are born with a spontaneous labour arrive after the due date. This is mainly because medical convention calculates the expected date of delivery from your last menstrual period rather than from actual moment of conception *(see p.27)*. Most doctors accept that anything up to 14 days after the expected date is normal.

Induction for "overdue" babies

Many units now offer induction at ten days after term and recommend it at 14 days after term because of the risk of late stillbirth. After 14 days, signs of postmaturity are carefully looked for. Screening involves monitoring the fetal heart and movements and ultrasound for amniotic fluid measurement.

However, waiting until the expected day of delivery is leaving it a bit late to face the prospect of an induced labour. This is something that should be discussed early in pregnancy and you and your doctor should try to agree on the best course.

Electronic fetal monitoring

Electronic fetal monitoring (EFM) is a method of recording the baby's heartbeat and your contractions during labour. It is the high-tech replacement for the ear trumpet or stethoscope, but has by no means superseded these. Some maternity units ask you to be monitored routinely for about 20 minutes, but if all is well there is no need for you to be continuously monitored throughout labour.

Monitoring is usually done with belts strapped around your abdomen that simultaneously pick up contractions and the baby's heartbeat, recording them on a graph. The print-out can then be interpreted by the midwife to make sure that the baby's heart is beating normally during the contraction. During a contraction, blood flow to your placenta is reduced for a few seconds and your baby's heart rate may dip. It then returns to normal when the contraction passes.

Occasionally, if the abdominal recording is of poor quality and your baby is thought to need constant monitoring, doctors may think it necessary to attach an electrode to the baby's scalp as well. The electrode is attached to his presenting part, usually to the skin on the top of his head, and provides an electrical contact that picks up his heartbeat. It is an accurate method of monitoring, but it does mean that your waters will have to be broken if they haven't already done so.

Electronic fetal monitoring involving a fetal scalp electrode used to confine mothers to bed, but nowadays it is less restricting. A method of monitoring by radio waves, known as telemetry, allows the mother to walk around away from the monitoring equipment. The electrode is still attached to the baby's head, but it is joined to a strap on the mother's thigh and not to a large machine. However, babies do suffer rashes where the electrode was clipped to them and there is no proof that they feel no pain when the clip is attached.

How monitoring can help

Electronic fetal monitoring provides the medical staff with a second-by-second report on the condition of your baby, so that they can intervene quickly if he is in

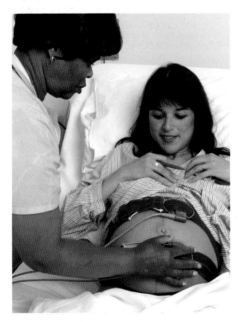

Monitoring in labour
Contractions are recorded by an external monitor strapped to your abdomen. An internal monitor is attached to your baby.

distress. If a doctor tells you that you need continuous EFM, try to see that as reassuring, because it will ensure that you get the best possible care for your baby.

Fetal monitor electrode

If your medical team think that your baby needs closer monitoring, they may want to attach an electrode to his head. Once your cervix is at least 2–3cm (¾–1¼in) dilated, you will be given an amniotomy to break your waters (see p.198) if they haven't broken already. An electrode is then attached to the part of the baby that is going to be born first, which is usually his head. The electrode pierces the skin slightly and provides an electrical contact that tracks the baby's heartbeat. Electronic signals are then relayed to the external monitor and a graph is printed out for the staff to interpret.

Continuous EFM

Monitoring the baby's heartbeat and the uterine contractions is essential if you are being induced (see p.197), if your labour is being accelerated or if you have an epidural, when you will be less able to feel the onset of contractions. Most hospitals now agree that continuous monitoring should be used routinely for mothers with a high risk of problems.

Obviously having a "window" into the uterus during labour is of great value, but machines can go wrong, and they need trained staff to use them correctly. If machines are incorrect, or interpreted incorrectly, this can lead to unnecessary intervention. Also, using a machine to monitor the baby may switch everyone's attention from the mother to the machine, which can be very upsetting for the woman who is in labour.

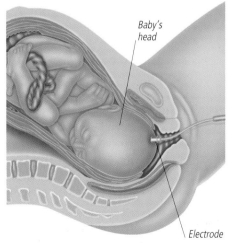

Baby's head

Electrode

Monitoring your baby
The electrode is attached to your baby's presenting part, usually his head. Many mothers do find EFM reassuring as they can watch their baby's heartbeat.

PROBLEMS WITH CONTINUOUS EFM

- The staff are more aware of any small changes and may therefore be more likely to intervene rather than letting labour take its natural course.
- Babies who are electronically monitored are three times more likely to be delivered by Caesarean section.
- EFM increases the electronic paraphernalia in the delivery room.
- Staff may be tempted to concentrate more on the machine than on the woman in labour.
- EFM may restrict movement, thus slowing down the labour and making fetal distress more likely.
- Attaching the electrode may bruise and hurt the baby's head.

17 Complications

Even the best planned labours may not go according to plan, especially for first-time mothers. You may become exhausted or your baby may become distressed and need to be delivered quickly. Thinking about the possibility of a forceps or Caesarean delivery in advance will help you to know what to expect should the situation arise.

Breech birth

A breech baby is one that is born buttocks first. Most babies move around freely until about the 32nd week of pregnancy when they turn head down (cephalic position). Four out of every hundred babies, however, stay put. If your baby is one of these, do not be concerned; most breech labours are smooth, though you will be advised to

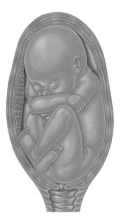

A well-flexed breech baby
It is possible to deliver a baby that is lying in this position vaginally, although you may need an episiotomy. Forceps may also be necessary.

have the baby in hospital. Doctors can try to turn breech babies by applying gentle external pressure on the abdomen.

Hospital birth is preferred
Attitudes towards breech births differ: some doctors feel that a breech baby should be delivered by Caesarean, others are less rigid. About 90 per cent are delivered by Caesarean in the UK.

Doctors do not generally recommend a home birth if your baby is in the breech position. However, if you are at home, try to adopt a supported upright position with your legs wide apart and your knees bent to give the baby's head more space.

After the birth, your genital region might be slightly swollen, but the swelling will subside within 48 hours. Because many breech births are helped by forceps, babies may have bruises on the face and head, but they will fade fast. You are more likely to have an episiotomy *(see p.195)* with a breech birth because the head has less time to be compressed during delivery.

BIRTH OF A BREECH BABY

The waters usually break early with a breech presentation and you'll probably feel contractions as bad backache (*see p.174*). Kneeling on all fours is a helpful position to relieve the discomfort during the first stage. For the birth, the supported squatting position is safest and an episiotomy may be done while you are in this position if necessary, although your doctor may prefer you to be lying down. Epidurals are advised to prevent you pushing before the cervix is fully dilated. If you then need a Caesarean section, this will save time and allow you to hold your baby the moment he is born.

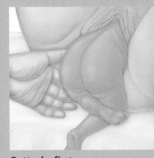 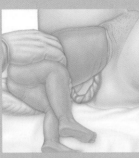 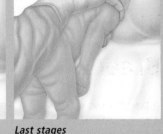

Buttocks first
A breech baby's buttocks press against the cervix and dilation occurs as with a head-down presentation. The buttocks are delivered first.

Delivery of the body
Once the baby's buttocks are clear of the birth opening, the body can be delivered. The body's weight will then start to pull the head down.

Last stages
In the final stages, the baby's arms emerge and his body is gently supported as his head is guided out. Sometimes forceps may be used.

Caesarean section

Inevitably there are slight risks, such as infection, bleeding and clot formation, associated with Caesarean section, as it is a major operation. There is also the disadvantage of being left with a scar on the uterus that may weaken it. The rate of Caesarean sections is still rising so there is some concern that the operation is being carried out without enough thought.

Caesarean sections are now usually done under an epidural or spinal anaesthetic (*see p.194*), which is safer than a general anaesthetic for you and the baby and means you can be conscious throughout. However, if an epidural isn't already in place at the time, an emergency Caesarean may have to be done under general anaesthetic.

You may know weeks or only days in advance that you are to have your baby by Caesarean section. This is known as a planned or "elective" Caesarean. You will be admitted to hospital on a certain day, but if you go into labour spontaneously beforehand, you will still be given a Caesarean. Some Caesareans need to be performed as emergencies if it's essential that the baby is delivered quickly.

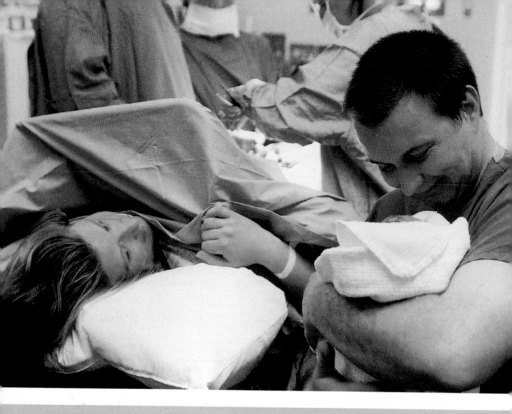

WHAT HAPPENS DURING A CAESAREAN

Some of your pubic hair will be shaved, the epidural anaesthesia will be set up (see p.194), you'll have an intravenous drip inserted into your arm so that fluids can be fed directly into your bloodstream, and a catheter will be inserted into your bladder to drain away urine. A screen will probably be placed in front of your face so you don't have to watch the operation. A Caesarean section usually takes about 45 minutes but the baby is delivered within the first 5–10 minutes. A small horizontal incision is made (*see left*) and the amniotic fluid is drained off by suction. The baby is then gently lifted out either by hand or with forceps. The cord is cut, the placenta is removed, and your uterus and abdomen are stitched. You and your partner can hold the baby while this third stage is completed. If everything is all right you can start nursing him as soon as possible. Depending on the reasons for the operation, your baby may be taken to special care for an observation period. The catheter and the drip will remain in for some hours and the stitches will be removed five days later.

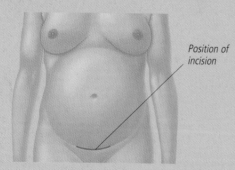

Position of incision

The horizontal line incision
The so-called "bikini line" incision is common for obvious cosmetic reasons and because the low transverse cut heals more effectively.

Having a Caesarean section
A screen is usually set up so that you can't see the operation taking place. Within 5–10 minutes of the incisions, the baby is delivered. Afterwards, your partner can hold the baby while you are stitched. You can nurse your baby as soon as you feel comfortable.

Preparing for a Caesarean

Some women find a Caesarean section a great disappointment after looking forward to a vaginal delivery. But the psychological effects can be minimized if you prepare yourself for having a Caesarean section and look on it as a positive experience.

Ask to see your obstetrician so that you and your partner can have a relaxed discussion about what the operation entails, what the procedures will be in the operating theatre, whether you can have epidural anaesthesia and be awake and alert during the operation, and whether your partner can be with you.

Ask your hospital clinic if there is a video available that shows what happens during a Caesarean. You can also prepare yourself by talking to other women who have had Caesarean sections. This is one of the best ways of preventing you from having negative feelings about it. Not only will you get moral support but you'll also get useful information about what it feels like, how long it takes to be completely fit again after the operation and tips on caring for your baby while your wound is healing. By talking to mothers who've had subsequent pregnancies after a Caesarean, you can allay your fears about the future. A self-help group will be able to put you in touch with midwives and obstetricians who have a flexible and realistic attitude to pregnancy after Caesarean section.

REASONS FOR A CAESAREAN SECTION

- Fetus shows signs of profound distress; this will be obvious if the heart rate slows or "dips" at each contraction and, more seriously, between contractions – this will show up on the printout from the electronic monitors (*see p.200*). If there is meconium in the amniotic fluid, the baby may have had a bowel movement which could indicate distress.
- The baby is extremely large or there may be cephalo-pelvic disproportion, where the baby's head is larger than the pelvic cavity.
- Breech babies (*see p.202*) are often delivered by Caesarean section, particularly in the United States, and increasingly in the UK.
- A previous baby was born by this method; this is the commonest reason for the operation in the United States.
- Prolapse of the umbilical cord through the cervix.
- Placenta praevia (*see p.156*).
- Placental abruption (*see p.156*).
- The baby needs to be delivered before term and induction and normal labour are considered to be an unnecessary risk to the baby or the mother.
- A serious infection of the vagina, such as a first-time attack of genital herpes.
- The cervix fails to dilate.
- Forceps fail to deliver the baby.
- Serious Rhesus incompatibility.

Some of the conditions that warrant abdominal delivery of the baby may not be apparent until labour has begun and this will then result in an emergency Caesarean section. Even so, many of these sections are now performed under epidurals and do not require general anaesthetic. An alternative is a spinal anaesthetic (which is like an epidural but cannot be topped up).

AFTER A CAESAREAN

When the operation is over you will return to the postnatal ward with your baby. Because you need plenty of rest after abdominal surgery, you can concentrate on feeding your baby and getting to know him. You will be expected to get up and move around the next day and you can start gentle exercises (*see p.228*) after two days. Most mothers feel normal from one week onwards after the operation. You will lose blood from the vagina just as you would after a vaginal delivery. Take care when lifting and avoid strenuous activity for at least six weeks. The scar will fade, usually in 3–6 months.

Lay baby on pillow to feed

Sitting up
When breast-feeding after a Caesarean section, your abdominal wound will be tender so bring your baby up to the level of your breast with pillows. Hold him with his feet under your arm.

Support wound with your hands

Lying down on your side
Place the baby on some pillows and then lower yourself down beside him to feed. You can support yourself on your elbow.

Standing up
Stand up perfectly straight when you get out of bed. When you cough or laugh, hold your hands over your wound to give yourself confidence. Keep moving around.

Vacuum extraction (ventouse)

The vacuum extractor, or ventouse, is a gentler alternative to forceps, except where the mother is unable to push. It takes up less room in the vagina than forceps and is easier to apply. It's used when there is a delay in the second stage of labour but where an easy delivery is ultimately anticipated. As for a forceps delivery the head does need to be in the birth canal.

There are few serious complications associated with vacuum extraction and there is much less potential for damage to the mother with vacuum extraction than with forceps. The process doesn't affect the shape of the baby's head. It does, however, leave a bruise, but this will fade within a week or two of the birth.

The cervix is almost always fully dilated for this procedure. A small metal or rubber cup connected to a vacuum apparatus is passed into the vagina and applied to the baby's head. The attached pump is then used to create a vacuum that makes the

plate or cup hold fast to the baby's head. This then becomes a "handle", which the obstetrician can use to rotate the baby's head and apply traction. By gentle pulling, and the mother's contractions, the baby's head is brought down into the pelvis and then slowly and gradually delivered.

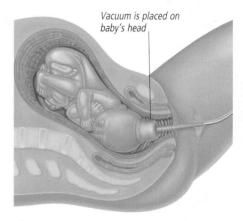

Vacuum is placed on baby's head

The vacuum extractor
A form of birth assistance, the vacuum extractor is mainly used in Europe; forceps are favoured in the US.

Forceps delivery

The decision to use forceps is a medical judgement on the part of your attendants. Forceps are only applied when the first stage is complete, the cervix is fully dilated, and the head is in the birth canal.

Forceps have saved the lives of many mothers and babies, and can reduce the need for a Caesarean for a baby that is stuck up in the pelvis. They are applied when your baby's head has descended into

your pelvis but fails to descend further; when a baby presents in a posterior position; in a breech delivery (*see p.202*); when the uterus fails to maintain contractions; and when you lack the strength to push. Occasionally, forceps may be used for a quick delivery early in the second stage if your baby shows signs of lacking oxygen, even if the birth is not imminent.

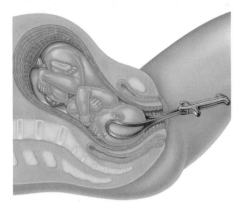

Forceps
These look like large sugar tongs and are designed to fit snugly over the sides of a baby's head, covering his ears. They're rather like a cage that protects the head from any pressure as it passes through the birth canal.

If you're going to have a forceps delivery, your legs will be put up in stirrups. A local anaesthetic will be injected into your perineum. Then the forceps will be inserted into your vagina one at a time. A few gentle pulls on the forceps, 30–40 seconds at a time, will bring your baby's head down on to your perineum. You should feel no pain. At this point you'll have an episiotomy (see p.195). Once your baby's head has been delivered, the forceps are removed and the rest of the body will be delivered as normal.

If longer forceps have to be used to pull the baby out, you may be given a pudendal nerve block. A spinal anaesthetic may also be used.

Prematurity and low birthweight

A baby born at less than 37 weeks is said to be premature, regardless of birthweight. A baby who weighs less than 2.5kg (5½lb) at term has a low birthweight. In either case the baby may need special care. The reason for a premature birth is not always known, but factors include pre-eclampsia (see p.160), multiple pregnancy (see p.157), premature rupture of the membranes and an abnormal placenta. Some maternal conditions, such as anaemia or malnutrition, and overwork, can also have an effect.

As a general rule, a premature labour begins without any warning and the first sign may be rupture of the membranes, the beginning of uterine contractions or vaginal bleeding. Provided it isn't too far advanced, attempts may be made to stop the labour so that the mother can be given

steroid injections to mature the fetal lungs and to reduce the work of breathing after the birth. The mother must be admitted to hospital and monitored closely. Usually a premature labour is shorter and easier than a full-term labour, mainly because the baby's head is smaller and softer than that of a full-term baby. Some premature births are accompanied by an episiotomy in order to protect the baby's soft head from pressure changes inside the birth canal.

The three most important aspects of a premature baby's health are his ability to breathe, feed and control his temperature. For these reasons the baby is nursed in a neonatal unit in an incubator where the temperature is controlled, where the oxygen supply can be easily changed according to the baby's needs, and where feeding can be achieved by a tube passed

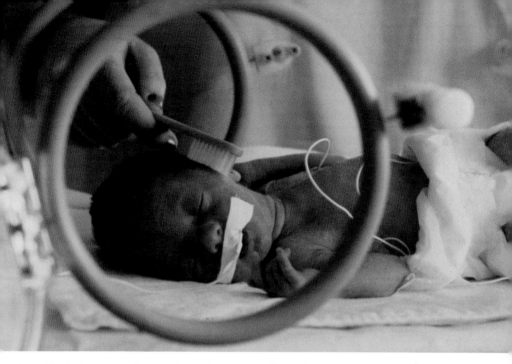

down the baby's nose. Because he will have poor resistance to infection, care is taken to keep equipment sterile.

If you are afraid that bonding may not take place, you can be reassured. You'll be encouraged to spend as much time as you can with your baby and to feed, touch and nurse him as soon as his condition allows. Until then you'll be able to watch the nurses caring for your baby. When your baby is ready, the staff will show you how

Getting to know your premature baby
Parents are encouraged to touch and care for their babies in the special-care baby unit.

to handle him safely. Breast milk can be particularly valuable for a premature baby, so express milk for him. This also helps to establish your milk supply, so that it's ready for him when he can suck. A very premature baby (24–30 weeks) may initially be fed intravenously with a special solution.

Newborn babies with jaundice

Jaundice is fairly common in newborn babies around about the third day of life. Medically it's called physiological jaundice, and it has no sinister connotations. A baby is born with a large number of red blood cells, which are rapidly broken down after it is born. When red blood cells break

down and are replaced, they release large quantities of the pigment known as bilirubin, which gives them their colour, and this has to be removed by the liver. At the time of birth a baby's liver is still immature and is not able to carry the excess load of bilirubin so the levels of pigments rise in the blood and give the skin a yellowish tinge. This type of jaundice usually fades at the end of the first week when the liver has cleared the blood of pigment. To help flush the excess bilirubin out of the baby's system, feed him often.

If bilirubin levels are high, the baby may be given light treatment (phototherapy). His eyes are covered and he's placed naked in a crib under an ultraviolet light. The light breaks down the bilirubin so that it can be passed more quickly by the baby in urine.

Postpartum haemorrhage

The uterus has a self-protecting device to stop it from bleeding after delivery. Once the fetus and the placenta have been expelled and the uterus is completely empty, it usually contracts down rapidly to about the size of a melon. This contraction closes the uterine arteries so that they cannot bleed. Under normal circumstances there's little bleeding after the delivery and little chance of infection.

In about 10 per cent of women, however, there is some bleeding after the birth, known as postpartum haemorrhage. The commonest cause is uterine atony – the uterus does not contract normally after delivery so the uterine arteries do not close as they should. It may also be caused by a fragment of placenta left in the uterus. This is usually diagnosed by examining the

placenta and finding that a portion is missing. In these cases the placenta is gently removed from the uterus.

If bleeding occurs more than 24 hours after delivery, the lochia (see p.219) may become bright red again. This can be caused by over-exertion, so your doctor will probably advise you to rest for several days. If the bleeding recurs or becomes heavy, this can mean infection or the retention of a small piece of placenta. Your doctor will probably prescribe antibiotics to cure the problem. If not, you may be referred back to the hospital. If you pass clots, call an ambulance immediately to take you to the nearest hospital, where the inner surface of your womb will be thoroughly but gently cleansed. If, however, the clots are due to infection, you'll need to take antibiotics.

Stillbirth

A baby is stillborn very rarely – it happens in fewer than one per hundred births. If the baby dies in the uterus before the 24th week of pregnancy the uterus usually goes spontaneously into labour within a day or so and a miscarriage will result. After 24

weeks the uterus may deliver the baby fairly quickly. Most, though not all, women are aware that something is wrong, because they have not felt any movements for 24 hours or more. No one knows quite why a baby should die in late pregnancy, but in most cases it is thought to be due to an insufficiently healthy placenta. The placenta may have failed to grow adequately or have become diseased in some way during the pregnancy so that it is no longer able to maintain an adequate oxygen and food supply to the baby. Occasionally the placenta begins to separate from the uterus (placental abruption – see p.156) and this can cause intrauterine death. Uncontrolled Rhesus incompatability (see p.160) or poorly stabilized diabetes can also lead to a stillbirth. When the baby dies, most of the sensations of being pregnant fade quite quickly as the levels of oestrogen and progesterone plummet. Even the uterus may diminish in size due to the absorption of the amniotic fluid from around the fetus. This may show up in the mother as dramatic weight loss. If a baby's death is suspected, an ultrasonic scan will be done to try to detect the fetal heartbeat. If the heart cannot be detected by the scan, it's unlikely that the baby is still alive.

Grieving is important

Because the baby is in a kind of cocoon inside the mother's body, its death does not adversely affect the mother's physical health. However, the emotional and psychological effects on both parents can be extremely traumatic. A woman will quite naturally feel all kinds of guilt, inadequacy, self-loathing, sadness and depression, and she may feel that she wants to withdraw and be completely by herself to come to terms with her grief. This can drive a wedge between her and her partner. You both need as much support as possible at this time, so for your own sakes, talk to each other about your feelings and confide in sympathetic friends and your doctor. It is also a good idea to seek bereavement counselling so that you can grieve fully and finally come to terms with your loss. Don't be surprised if this takes some time, even several months, but look forward to the future; most couples who have lost a baby do eventually become proud parents of healthy babies.

Delivery of the baby

Until recently it was thought that labour should be allowed to start spontaneously – it usually begins within two or three days of the baby's death – and should not be interfered with. Most women find that they want to deliver the baby as soon as possible after death has been confirmed, and in any case, labour is induced quickly to avoid the possibility of infection. Delivery of a stillborn baby by Caesarean is not recommended because of the risks of surgery, but there are no barriers to pain relief for a woman in this situation.

Many parents who have experienced a stillbirth find that touching, holding and naming their baby help them to come to terms with the loss. It also helps to have a photograph of the baby and to hold a proper funeral to say goodbye. The hospital will help you with the arrangements if you wish or you can make your own with a local funeral director. Ask your doctor to explain the reasons for your loss, but accept that no one may know exactly why your baby died. You may find that it helps to get in touch with others who have suffered such a bereavement (see p.243) – their experience can help you to understand your own reactions.

18 The first days

The birth of your baby is a climax to the nine months of waiting and anything that follows must, to a certain extent, fall in its shadow. During the first three days while you're waiting for the milk to come in, you may feel excited or tentative or you may find yourself in a state of shock. It's thrilling to explore your new baby and to enjoy quiet moments together, but don't be surprised if at times it feels like a bit of a let-down.

Becoming a mother

Immediately after the birth you'll probably be tired, but many women feel elated and full of energy. Everyone reacts differently. If you're in hospital there will be the ward routines to deal with, but once you're home, you can enjoy the peace and security of familiar surroundings, and get to know your baby. Life for the next few weeks will revolve around the baby, but in time both of you, together with your partner and any other children should begin to adjust to a more settled routine.

Your baby's appearance
At last your new baby is born, a completely new human being with his own unique personality and appearance.

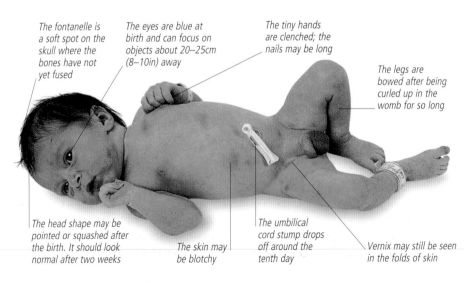

The fontanelle is a soft spot on the skull where the bones have not yet fused

The eyes are blue at birth and can focus on objects about 20–25cm (8–10in) away

The tiny hands are clenched; the nails may be long

The legs are bowed after being curled up in the womb for so long

The head shape may be pointed or squashed after the birth. It should look normal after two weeks

The skin may be blotchy

The umbilical cord stump drops off around the tenth day

Vernix may still be seen in the folds of skin

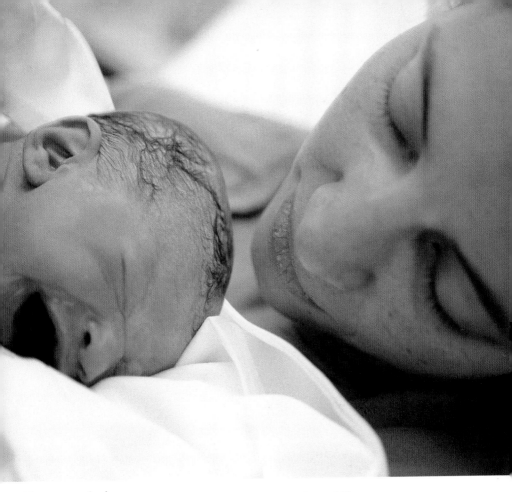

Your new baby

At birth, your baby may have lots of hair, or be quite bald. She may not look quite as you expected, but as the days go by any marks or bruising from the birth will fade. The content of your baby's first bowel movement after birth is called meconium, a dark, greenish, sticky substance. This will change gradually to more normal bowel movements once feeding starts.

Immediately after birth, your baby will be tested and given an Apgar score (*see p.214*); this is an indication of her general well-being. Later on she'll be weighed and measured; your midwife will continue to

The first hour of life
The sooner you start to touch and cuddle your baby the better for the bonding process, and you'll help her adapt to her new world.

do this regularly for the first ten days. The doctor will give your baby a general examination to check for abnormalities and her hearing will be checked.

Around the sixth day after the birth, a blood sample is taken from your baby's heel. This checks for PKU (phenylketonuria) and congenital hypothyroidism, both of which are rare causes of mental disability that can be treated if detected.

NEWBORN REFLEXES

Babies are born with certain reflexes that help them to survive the first days outside the womb. For example, babies put to the breast immediately after delivery will root for the nipple and suck. These reflexes gradually fade over the coming weeks as the baby learns new skills.

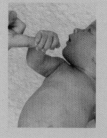

Stepping
A newborn baby will make these movements if you hold her under the arms and let her feet touch a firm surface. This doesn't mean that she will walk early; she will have to learn that technique later on.

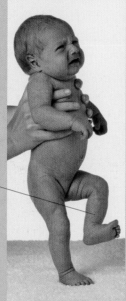

Leg movements

Grasping
If you place your finger in the palm of your baby's hand, she will grasp it tightly. The grasp is so strong that her whole weight can be supported if she grasps your fingers with both hands. The soles of her feet also curl over if touched.

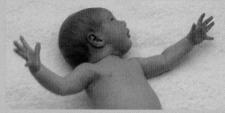

Moro reflex
If your baby is startled she will throw out her arms and legs as if to catch hold of something. Her limbs will then curl in towards her body and her fists will clench.

THE APGAR SCALE

When your baby is born, her condition is assessed according to a series of standard tests at one and five minutes. Each test is given a score of 2, 1 or 0.

A score of 7 or over is normal, as is a low first score with a normal second score. A low second score may mean she needs the attention of the paediatrician.

SIGN	2 POINTS	1 POINT	0 POINTS
Heart rate	above 100 beats per minute	below 100 beats per minute	absent
Breathing	regular	irregular	absent
Movements	active	some	limp
Skin colour	pink	bluish extremities	blue
Reflex response	cries	whimpers	absent

Bonding with your new baby

It's difficult to describe what bonding is; it's certainly getting to know your baby and exploring her with your eyes, nose, ears, fingertips and mouth, and even your tongue. It's also to do with attachment, protectiveness and possessiveness. This early attachment is possibly the strongest bond between human beings, and necessarily so, as it ensures the nurturing of infants, and hence the survival of the human race.

First contact

Establishing a relationship with your baby begins the second she is born. If possible you should be left in private with your partner with a minimum of interruption for some time during the first hour after the birth. Research has shown that babies are usually quiet, but very alert, in the first hour of life, and in this state they are extremely responsive. They will stare intently at your face if held 20–25cm (8–10in) away. They can focus their eyes at this distance and respond to the human face.

In addition, like most newborn animals, human babies have an instinct to bond with their parents. This is the right time for attachment to a caring adult, so both of you should make the most of it. Keep the lighting low and lay your baby against your body so that you make skin-to-skin contact. Looking into your baby's eyes renders her a person and not a thing, and skin contact allows you to feel each other as warm human beings.

The midwife may want to stitch you at this time, because early stitching is quicker and easier than if left until later, when the tissues may be swollen. It will probably be possible to hold your baby while it is being done or else your partner can have valuable one-to-one contact with his new baby. Other cleaning up can wait a while.

Benefits to you

All aspects of the bonding process – your voice, smell, touch, caresses, fondling – are good for your baby, and they're also good for you. The sooner you touch and fondle your baby, the more quickly your bleeding will cease, the more strongly your uterus contracts down and the more effectively your breasts will respond with the let-down of colostrum (see p.221) and later milk. You'll also be increasing your confidence in handling the baby and helping her adapt to a new environment.

First feed

Studies show that babies adapt more easily when they are held, soothed, crooned at and allowed to feed at will. Soon after you take hold of your baby, try putting her to your breast. Touch her cheek with your nipple and she will turn towards the breast. If she shows little perseverance – she may be sleepy if you had drugs for pain relief – express a little colostrum onto her lips to encourage her. Your partner can help at this point by supporting the baby's head until you feel comfortable.

You may not bond instantly, however, particularly if you had a long or difficult labour. Don't worry; you have plenty of time to get to know your baby later.

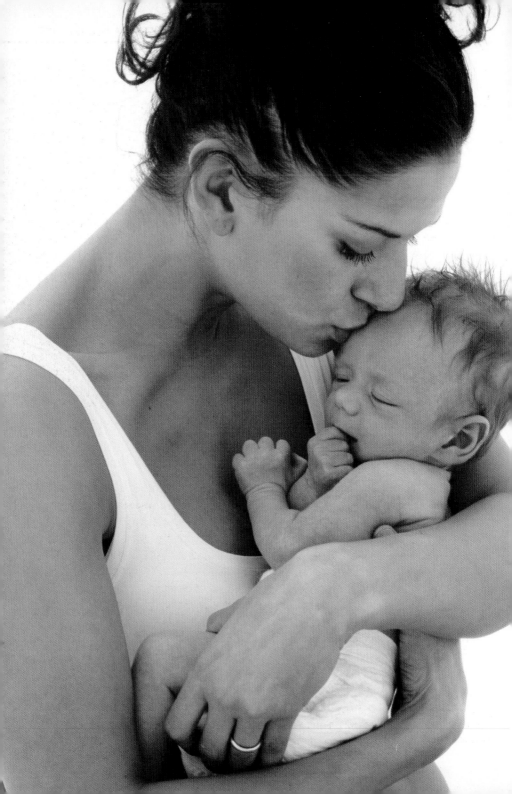

Importance of bonding

If it seems that I'm emphasizing this bonding process, I feel it's for good reason. Research has shown that parents who are given unrestricted contact with their children immediately after delivery rear their children in a more constructive way. They are more sympathetic to problems, ask more questions, give reasons for their actions and explain situations more readily than do parents whose babies are taken away at birth. A further part of this research showed that at the age of five years the children who had had extended contact with their parents scored higher in intelligence tests than the control group. This does not mean that good bonding with your infant makes your baby a more intelligent child. What I think it points to is that it makes you a different kind of parent and possibly a better one.

FATHER'S FIRST CONTACT

Paternal bonding with an infant is not very different and certainly just as important as maternal bonding. So during this sensitive period after the birth it's important for you to hold your baby and make eye and skin contact. If you have been present at the birth and comforted your partner throughout the labour, this is a good beginning. Stay with your partner and your baby as long as possible after the birth. Be responsive to the cues that your infant will give you.

It may take you a little longer and you may have to fit yourself into the role to achieve the same degree of responsiveness as the mother. All this can be helped by early and extended contact with your baby in her first weeks of life. Very often the birth of a child helps a man to express and enjoy emotions that society primes him to repress.

Establishing a routine

The first few days will be hard; labour and birth are physically and emotionally draining. If you are in hospital you are subject to a certain amount of routine – regular checks by midwives, ward rounds by obstetricians or paediatricians, meals at certain times, visits by physiotherapists, family and friends, and so on – plus learning to feed, change and bath your baby. I had my first baby in hospital and

Early days
Your baby may seem very vulnerable in the first weeks, but don't worry – she's equipped with reflexes and behaviour that help her survive.

expected to have a restful time; instead I hardly had a minute to myself and was utterly exhausted at night – I couldn't wait to get home to peace and security.

Even if you have your baby at home, you'll find that one activity succeeds another almost without respite, and all the time you are learning. You may have read all the baby books that are available, but no book tells you about your baby. There's no short cut to learning about your baby's care because you have to take your lead from her. Babies don't know night from day and they require the same attention during the night as they do during the day.

The smaller your baby, the more often you will have to feed her. Small babies, say 3.1kg (7lb) or under, require food at least every four hours and often there may be only three hours or two and a half hours between feeds. You should feed on demand; if you do, your baby will find her own routine faster than if you try to impose your routine on her. At least twice during the night your newborn baby will need a feed and a nappy change. Nearly everyone I have spoken to seems to have had a well-behaved baby who slept for six hours during the night within a week of being delivered. Well, mine didn't! The baby that gives you more than four hours' sleep during the night is an exception.

Respond to the baby's needs

The best way to manage all that's demanded of you and to stay cheerful and get enough rest is to take your cue from your baby. You're going to have to learn to catnap because the only chance you may get to sleep during the first few days is when your baby is asleep. Just after delivery you have little stamina and will easily become exhausted from physical effort. Emotionally you are in a vulnerable state because of the sudden withdrawal of pregnancy hormones. Little problems seem insurmountable and big ones insoluble. You may feel short-tempered and irritable with flashes of elation in between. You may be tearful as soon as anything goes wrong and the next minute find yourself imbued with strong resolutions. Don't expect too much of yourself.

Once you are home don't worry about day-to-day domestic chores. Let them pile up; any outside helper can see to those

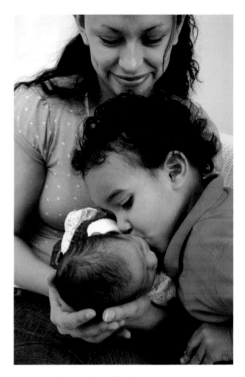

New member of the family
When you introduce your new baby to an older child, let him feel and touch her.

things. Save your energy to concentrate on what matters, and there really are only a few things that should get top priority: the baby, then you, then your partner and any other children, then all of you as a family unit. Be unscrupulous in asking for help, even if it's only for the first week, so that you have time on your own to get to know your baby and look after her needs.

Most newborn babies have the same basic needs in the first few weeks of life, and once you've established a routine, you can then set about deciding what your needs are and how best to organize yourself on a typical day.

The mother

You may be dismayed at your new post-pregnant shape. Your stomach will have sagged, your breasts will look large and your thighs will seem heavy. Don't let it get you down: start on your postnatal exercises *(see p.228)* right away.

Afterpains

Throughout our fertile lives the uterus never stops contracting; these contractions are felt as menstrual cramps at the time of our periods, as Braxton Hicks contractions throughout pregnancy, and after delivery as afterpains. Uterine contractions after delivery are stronger and more painful than usual because they are the means by which the uterus contracts down to its former non-pregnant size. The faster and harder it contracts down the less likelihood there is of any postpartum haemorrhage *(see p.210)*. The contractions are usually not severe with the first baby, but subsequently women become more conscious of them. They are more severe in breast-feeding women, but are an excellent sign that you are getting back to normal quickly. They usually disappear after three or four days.

Lochia

For anything up to six weeks you may pass lochia, which is a discharge of blood and mucus from the uterus. Immediately after delivery it is like a pink or red menstrual flow and after a few days it becomes a dark brown. It gradually fades to a creamy colour and finally becomes white. Use sanitary pads as protection and avoid tampons until after your first full period.

Bowels and bladder

Use the toilet as soon as you possibly can after delivery. You may not want to pass a bowel motion for 24 hours or more. Don't worry about this, but obey the first call to move your bowels and take care not to strain. Drinking water and walking about will help to get your bowels working. There may be some hesitancy before the urine starts to flow. This is nothing to worry about and is usually the result of swelling of the perineum and the tissues that surround the bladder and the urethral opening. A good way to get started is to sit in some warm water, try out the Kegel exercises *(see pp.122–123)*, and pass urine into the water. This is not unhygienic if you wash yourself thoroughly afterwards. If you've had stitches, passing urine may sting. Try pouring warm water over yourself as you are passing urine to reduce stinging.

You may also notice an increase in the amount of urine passed for the first few days. This is the way your body eliminates the excess fluid you have accumulated during your pregnancy.

COPING WITH STITCHES

Most stitches dissolve after five or six days. If you are bruised or the stitches cause you discomfort:
- Sit on an inflatable rubber ring.
- After bathing, dry the area thoroughly with a hair dryer rather than a towel.
- Put salt in the bath to aid healing.
- Hold a clean pad against the stitches when you move your bowels.
- Don't get constipated *(see p.146)*.

Feeding

Whichever method of feeding you choose, remember the colostrum in your breasts during the first three days contains valuable antibodies that will protect your baby against all kinds of diseases.

Breast-feeding

This is something that you have to learn for yourself – no one can give you any lessons. If you are in hospital, ask the nursing staff to help you to get started. Establishing breast-feeding is always easier if you put the baby to the breast within a few minutes of delivery (*see p.215*). Once you've achieved successful suckling in the happy relaxed atmosphere that surrounds the birth, you'll feel confident about future feeding. If this isn't possible, start feeding as soon as you can and try to relax and enjoy the experience. You may feel sore around the nipples, or your baby may not be very good at feeding at first, but it will come in time. Remember every woman is equipped to feed her baby, and no breast is too small to feed a baby. Supply automatically meets demand.

SUCCESSFUL BREAST-FEEDING

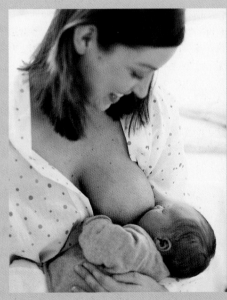

Rooting reflex
If you touch the baby's cheek with your nipple or finger, she'll turn to the breast and try to latch on. This is known as the rooting reflex. It is instinctive and can be encouraged if you express colostrum onto her lips.

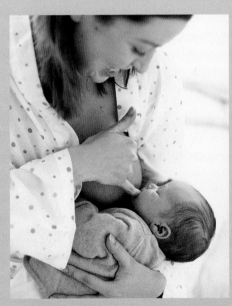

Breaking the suction
At the end of a feed don't pull your breast away from the baby. This will make your nipple sore. Instead insert your finger into the corner of her mouth and gently ease her off the breast, or press down on her chin.

Colostrum

During the first three days the breasts produce light, yellow-coloured colostrum. It is a perfect food for the first days of your baby's life. It contains water, protein and minerals in just the right proportion to take care of all your baby's nutritional needs. Colostrum also contains valuable antibodies that protect your baby against diseases to which you've developed a resistance, such as polio and influenza. Besides all that, it contains a laxative that gets your newborn baby's bowels in motion. After about 72 hours, colostrum is replaced by breast-milk, and for about two to three days, your breasts will feel heavy and full.

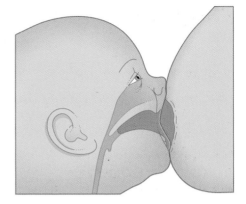

Latching on
The baby is properly latched on when she has the whole of the nipple area in her mouth, with her tongue underneath the nipple. She presses the top of her mouth against the milk reservoirs.

Let-down reflex

This is the automatic reaction by which the body makes milk available in the breasts. The reflex is a complicated chemical chain reaction that occurs in seconds and is set off either upon stimulation of your nipple by the baby, or by your baby's hunger cry or even by the thought of your baby. At this trigger the pituitary gland releases a hormone, oxytocin, which causes the milk-producing cells to empty their milk into the reservoirs in the nipple area. If you are not ready to feed, press the sides of your breasts firmly to control the flow.

Getting breast-feeding going

In the first days the nipples are delicate and they need time to toughen up so increase the length of time on each breast gradually. Two minutes on each breast will give your baby sufficient colostrum at first. Make sure she is properly latched on (see below). Build up the time on each breast to 10 minutes on each side by the time the milk has come in on about the third or fourth day, but don't try to stick to a timetable. Babies suck most strongly in the first five minutes, during which they take about 80 per cent of the feed. When she has had enough, she'll lose interest and start to play with your breast. She may turn away and fall asleep. You'll know if she hasn't had enough because she will wake hungry and cry. At the next feed, alternate the breast you start on.

Breast care

You'll need to take care of your breasts during the early days. Buy at least two of the best maternity bras you can afford *(see p.135)* and pay strict attention to the daily hygiene of your breasts and nipples. Bathe them every day with water; don't use soap because it dehydrates the skin and can encourage a crack or a sore to develop. Always handle your breasts with care. Never rub them dry, always pat dry.

After feeding, if possible, leave your nipples open to the air for a short time. Wear pads inside your bra to soak up any milk that may leak, and change these pads often. Don't leave a wet pad in contact with your breast for any length of time. If one of your nipples becomes sore, put a drop of camomile or calendula cream on the nipple two or three times a day.

Help with breast-feeding

Give yourself time to prepare for feeding. Have a comfortable chair ready, and surround yourself with everything you need. Keep some water beside you. If you're in bed, prop yourself up with pillows.

- Support your baby along the length of her back and use your hand and fingers to support the back of her neck to bring her up to your breast. She should be able to reach your nipple without effort. Support your back and arms with pillows and place a pillow on your lap to raise and provide extra support to your baby if necessary.

WINDING AND POSSETING

Some babies swallow enough air during feeding to cause them discomfort, and their piercing screams after a feed are silenced as soon as the wind is passed. Other babies are never bothered by wind. If you aren't sure, hold your baby in a upright position and pat her back. If nothing happens, and the baby is happy, there is no need to wait for a burp. Your baby may regurgitate (posset) a little milk when she burps. Some babies posset, others don't. The commonest cause is overfeeding, and there is nothing to worry about even if it looks a lot. Have a muslin cloth ready or put a bib on the baby to catch the posset.

- Relax your shoulders. If you have to bend your back to lower the nipple to the baby, you will quickly become tired and your neck and shoulders will tense up.
- If your breasts become full of milk soon after a feed, express a little (see p.236) to help you to feel more comfortable.
- If your breasts are full and hard, the nipple will flatten out and your baby will have difficulty latching on. Express a little milk before feeding to soften the areola and as the milk flows the baby will latch on and suck.
- If you get too tired, you can express some milk and put it in a bottle for your partner or a friend to give to the baby.
- To ease engorgement, apply hot or cold cloths to your breasts and with gentle massage the milk will flow.
- If you develop a crack, express from the sore breast until the skin heals. Give the baby the expressed milk from a sterilized spoon if you don't want to bother with bottles.
- If your baby refuses the breast it may be because she is having difficulty in breathing. Press down on the top of your breast gently with a finger to clear a space for her nostrils.
- If you feel feverish and notice a shiny, red patch on your breast, consult your doctor. This could be a blocked duct.

Bottle-feeding

If you've decided to bottle-feed your baby, you'll experience about two uncomfortable days while the milk dries up in your breasts. You'll be advised to wear a good, firm bra and to take mild analgesics if necessary to relieve the pain of engorgement. By the fifth day after your baby's birth, your

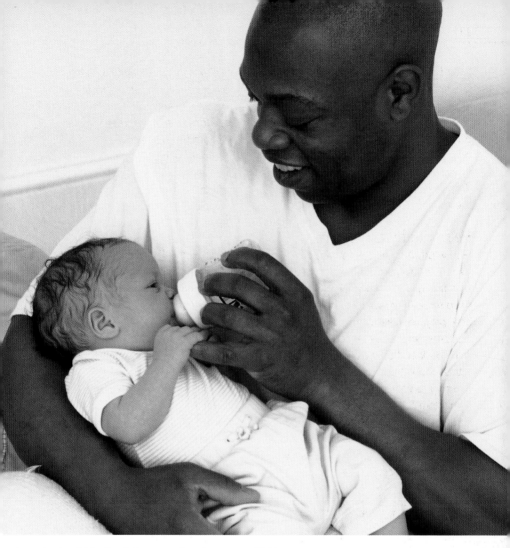

breasts should be back to normal and much more comfortable.

The main advantage of bottle-feeding is that the new father can be involved right from the beginning with feeding and feeding-time activities. When either of you feeds your baby, make sure your back is supported and hold the bottle firmly at an angle so that the teat is always full of milk. If not, the baby will suck in air with her feed. The teat should be well back in the baby's mouth. If your baby shows no

Making eye contact
Whether bottle-feeding or breast-feeding, always hold your baby so that she can see your face.

interest in feeding, encourage her to "root" (*see p.220*) for the bottle by gently touching her cheek with your finger or the teat. If the teat suddenly goes flat, release the vacuum by gently pulling on the bottle, to allow the milk to flow again. Sometimes the teat becomes blocked. If this happens change it for a new, sterile one.

Bathing and changing

Until your baby is six weeks old, the only parts that need daily bathing are her head, hands and bottom. To do this you need to "top and tail" her everyday. You can also give your baby a bath but you don't need to do this everyday. Try to wash your baby at about the same time every day so that you can both establish a routine.

them as your hands will be full.
• Undress her to her vest and nappy. Wipe her face and hands (*see below*). Wrap her in a towel, then wash and dry her hair. Finally undress her ready for the bath. Play with her in the bath. Wrap her in a warm dry towel after the bath and dress her again.

Giving your baby a bath
• Warm the room to at least 20°C (68°F) and use water that is about 32°C (90°F); it should be warm and not hot when you dip your wrist or elbow into it.
• Don't use soap to wash your baby as it dehydrates the skin.
• Try to bath your baby at a time when you will not be disturbed. Have everything you need – towels, new nappy and clothes – ready before you start, otherwise you won't be able to reach

Reusable or disposable nappies?
There are many issues that you'll have to think about when you are deciding which nappies to use. Your first choice in nappies will be between resuable fabric and disposable types. Disposable nappies make nappy changing as simple as it can be. They are easy to put on and can be discarded when they are wet or dirty. You can buy sizes ranging from newborn to toddler and there are special styles for boys and girls. They are convenient when you're

TOPPING AND TAILING

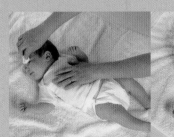
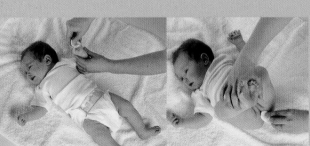

1 Fill a bowl with warm, boiled water. Wipe each eye with separate piece of cotton wool dipped in the water and squeezed dry. Always wipe from the inner side of the eye outwards.

2 Using fresh cotton wool, wipe around her neck, behind her ears, her face, mouth and nostrils. Don't clean inside her ears. Pat her dry with a soft towel and wipe her hands and arms with a facecloth.

3 Put on a new vest, then remove her nappy. With a new piece of cotton wool, wipe all around the genital area. Dry her skin well. Most babies enjoy the freedom of not having a nappy on for a time.

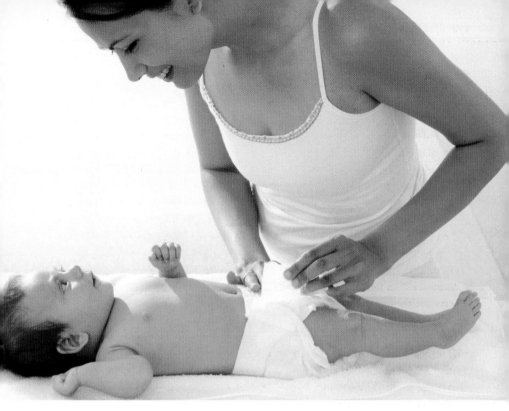

travelling as you need fewer nappies and less space to change in, and you don't have to carry wet, smelly nappies home with you to be washed. But millions of these nappies are now thrown away each day and they are creating a waste problem.

Many parents prefer to use disposables, although an increasing debate on the environmental issues has led many parents to reconsider the virtues of reusable nappies. Although initially more expensive to buy than disposables, reusable nappies work out cheaper as you can use them over and over again and for more than one child. Also you can buy shaped nappies that are as easy to use as disposables.

Yet the issue is not clear cut: the detergents required to clean fabric nappies can be viewed as pollutants to the water supply, and the energy required to wash

Changing time
Nappy changing need not be a chore. You can use it as a time when you play and talk to your baby on a one-to-one basis.

them might also be regarded as wasteful. While reusable nappies are cheaper than disposables in the long run, you need to consider the electricity bills for frequent washing-machine runs, and the cost in your time. Bear in mind that there are now nappy-laundering services in many areas.

What is clear is that providing that the nappy is changed as frequently as necessary, and that the basic rules of hygiene are observed, your baby will be happy whatever you choose. The general techniques for cleaning and caring for your baby's bottom are the same whatever kind of nappy you choose.

Postnatal blues

Weepiness and depression are common around the third or fourth day when your milk starts to flow. If you find that your depression is more than just feeling a bit low and it lasts longer than two weeks, you should seek medical help immediately. Don't allow the depression to drag on thinking that it will disappear. Early medical help may defuse the situation, and going without help may worsen your depression and it will take longer for you to feel better.

Change in hormone levels

Like any other depression, postnatal depression is more likely the wider the disparity between expectations and reality. Any negative feelings you may have, whether it is about yourself or the baby or about motherhood, will be exaggerated in the early days because of the fragile emotional state you are in. It's the fault of your hormones which, after having been at very high levels for nine months, are suddenly plunged back to the comparatively low levels of normality. This enormous swing renders most women tearful, weepy, irritable, indecisive, moody, uncommunicative, anxious, insomniac and depressed. After the initial euphoria has worn off, reality seems difficult to cope with. You'd be absolutely wrong to think that the early days are easy. They are not. You'd be wrong to think that you have a lead on every woman and know how to manage the early days. No one does. The expertise, the tricks, the responsibilities of motherhood are acquired only through learning, which takes time, so be easy on yourself. Gather as much information as you can, talk to the midwife, the health visitor, the doctor, to friends who have had babies and to experienced mothers.

Don't try to keep up appearances. Let everybody but the baby and your partner fend for themselves. Be as open as your personality allows you to be. Consult your partner and friends about worries and problems. One of the best ways to keep the stresses, strains and new responsibilities of motherhood in perspective and prevent them escalating into a serious emotional disturbance is to talk.

Rest and sleep

Sufficient rest and sleep in the first few days are essential although difficult to achieve. Many women feel exhausted after childbirth; it seems that your body is letting you down because it simply cannot function the way it did before you were

---

GETTING ENOUGH REST

- Never ignore signs of tiredness. Stop whatever you are doing, if it isn't essential, and lie down with your feet raised slightly above your head.
- You don't have to go to sleep to conserve your strength; resting will give your heart, lungs and other vital organs time to recover.
- Whether you've had a hospital or a home birth, enlist someone to help with the household chores and the baby so that you can rest during the day.
- Discourage visitors if you feel unable to cope. Put yourself and the baby first and ask to be left alone.

pregnant. One of the reasons why you feel so exhausted is that the volume of your blood has been suddenly cut by 30 per cent. Therefore a sufficient volume of blood cannot reach your muscles for them to work efficiently and so they feel weak and tire easily. It will take you several weeks to readjust to this enormous change.

I well remember going shopping five days after delivery to get a few things for the baby. I didn't have to walk far to the shops and I wasn't carrying anything heavy, but before I got back to my car, I had to sit down and rest. This is normal and you should try to avoid even moderate activity.

Mother-love
Everyone thinks that mother-love comes ready-made with breast-milk. This is not so. Many women would admit that they feel very little in terms of deep love for their baby within the first 24 to 48 hours. Love has to grow and the bonding process takes time. There is nothing wrong with you if it takes several days or even a couple of weeks. Mother-love is not something that can be pre-arranged, and feelings of caring, protectiveness and love for your new baby have to develop in their own time.

Coping with being in hospital
You may find life in hospital tiring and difficult, but most women don't stay in for long these days. On the other hand there are things to enjoy. You'll have company and can share your experiences and worries with other new mothers. A pleasant social life can develop between mothers with new babies and you may form friendships that last well after confinement. The companionship and friendliness that exist between mothers in maternity wards can be very comforting.

If ward life doesn't suit you, do tell the nursing staff. There are many ward sisters who take an enlightened and flexible view and will do their best to help you. If this isn't possible, you will find that your unhappiness deepens. It would be sad if the first few days with your baby were marred by the frustrations of hospital life, so it would probably be better for all concerned if you asked for a discharge from hospital and, if necessary, discharged yourself. If you don't feel strong enough to make a decision like this, ask your partner to help you. Provided you and your baby are well there's normally no reason why you would not be able to go home.

LEAVING HOSPITAL

Hospital practice varies, but whether you leave hospital after 12 hours or a few days, some of the following procedures will apply to your discharge.
- A doctor or midwife will check that your uterus is returning to its pre-pregnant size and that your stitches are healing. The lochia will be inspected to see if you've passed any blood clots.
- You'll be asked about contraception, and given a prescription if you need one. A low-dose pill may be prescribed (see p.235) if you're breast-feeding.
- The midwife will show you how to clean your baby's umbilical cord.
- Your baby will be checked by a paediatrician; if you have any worries, ask now. You will be advised to take your baby to a clinic for a six-week developmental check-up.
- You'll be given a date for your postnatal check-up or advised to see your doctor near to that date.

Postnatal exercises

Exercise at least once a day as soon as you can after delivery. It's best to exercise for a short time, say five minutes, several times a day. Lie on your stomach for the first few days too, to help bring the uterus forwards into its pre-pregnant position.

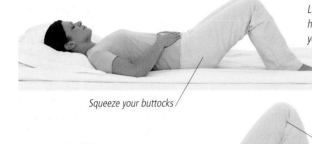

Squeeze your buttocks

Bend one knee

Stomach muscles
Lie flat with your knees bent and your hands on your stomach. Squeeze your buttocks together and press your back into the bed. Hold and relax. Practise your pelvic floor exercises at the same time (see p.123).

Foot pedalling
Flex your foot up and down as if you were pedalling. This is one of the first exercises you can do after delivery. It encourages good circulation and prevents your ankles and feet from swelling.

Hip hitching
Lie on your back, bend one knee and flex the foot of the straight leg. Lengthen that straight leg by pushing your heel away from you. Then shorten it by bringing it up towards you (without bending your knee). Make sure you don't arch your back.

Curl-ups
Lie on your back, with your knees bent. With your hands placed lightly on your thighs, slowly raise your head and shoulders and reach for your knees with your hands.

Reach for your knees

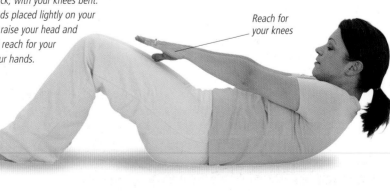

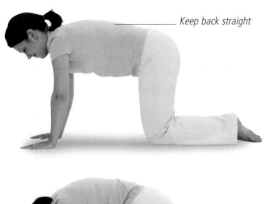

Keep back straight

PELVIC FLOOR TEST

When your baby is about three months old, test your pelvic floor muscles. Jump up in the air with your legs apart and cough hard. If there is a leakage of urine, practise your pelvic floor exercises more often (*see p.123*). See your doctor if there is no improvement by six months.

Take knee to forehead

Cat arching
Kneel down on all fours with your hands directly beneath your shoulders (top). Keep your back straight. Bend one leg up and try to touch your knee with your forehead (centre). Stretch the leg out behind you, elongate your neck to make a straight line from head to toe. Hold for a few seconds (bottom). Repeat with other leg.

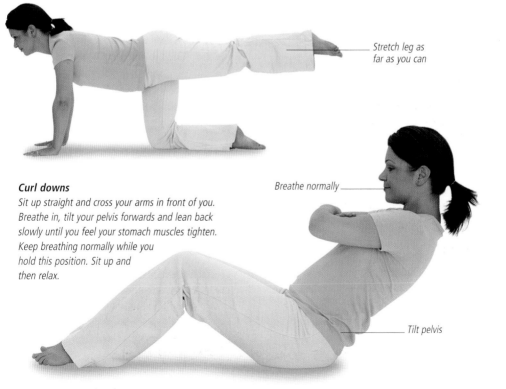

Stretch leg as far as you can

Breathe normally

Tilt pelvis

Curl downs
Sit up straight and cross your arms in front of you. Breathe in, tilt your pelvis forwards and lean back slowly until you feel your stomach muscles tighten. Keep breathing normally while you hold this position. Sit up and then relax.

19 Getting back to normal

Every woman feels differently after the birth of her baby. Some women want to cocoon at home, taking their time to get used to motherhood in private. Others choose to throw themselves into socializing and join mother-and-baby groups as soon as they can. But do give yourself at least seven to ten days to build up strength before you get back to normal routines. Being back home is comforting, but as time goes on, if you don't make plans to meet people, you may feel isolated. However, motherhood could open many doors to you. You'll find that getting out and about with your baby can create a new way of life within your local community.

The new family

How much you and your baby will have established a routine depends largely on how long you stayed in hospital. A stay of three to five days allows you to get to know each other and, taking the lead from your baby, you will have probably formed a loose timetable to suit his needs.

On the other hand, if you leave hospital within the first day or two after delivery or if you had a home birth, your routines will be based on the day-to-day running of the household. There has to be give and take on both sides; the baby is an important member of the household, but he also has to fit in with other members of the family and their needs. There's no question in my mind, that the quickest way to establish a routine is to let your baby lead you and to organize yourself, your life and your interests into the time that he leaves you

free to do so, after you have taken care of all his needs. It's easiest on the whole household if you wait and see how often the baby wants to feed, how often he wants to sleep, when his usual waking times and sleeping times are. Then try to dovetail your chores around his clock.

Rest when you can

One of the most important things for you to note is your baby's longest sleeping time. Try to fit in a nap or a rest during the same time. Establishing a routine does not mean "training" your baby to eat, sleep and play according to a timetable that suits you. What it really means is feeding and playing with your baby when he's awake, and trying to rest when he's asleep.

One of the early ways to introduce the baby to a diurnal rhythm is to make night

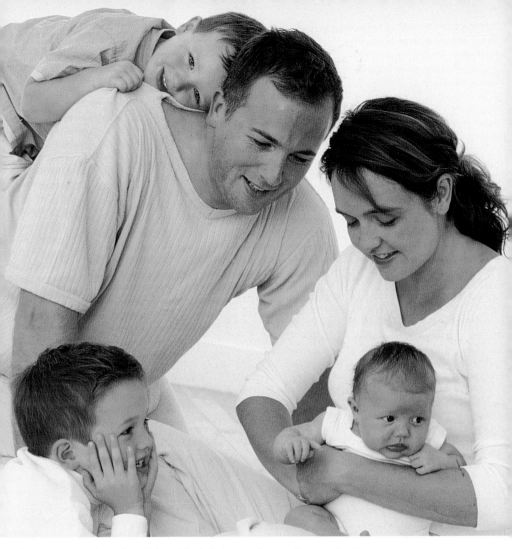

feeds quiet and in a low light with as little disruption as possible. The daylight hours will then become synonymous in his mind with bustle and noise.

Relationship with your partner

With a new baby, a mother starts out on an exciting relationship with another person and may feel little sense of loss if the closeness with her partner gradually diminishes. This is not so for a father and a woman should remember this. A man's

Integrating your family
Closeness and involvement as a family will help your older children to accept the new baby without feeling shut out of your world.

jealousy of his baby is not uncommon and many men confess to feeling pushed out by the baby and neglected by their partners. You must make sure that both of you understand that it is inevitable in the early days for the baby to become the main focus of attention. Therefore you should both make time for each other. One way to resume your closeness is to take a nap together at the end of the working day.

One adjustment you both have to make is that your life can't be as spontaneous as it was before the baby. You both need to become more flexible and possibly more tolerant than you were before, ready to give time and attention to each other when the opportunity arises. Look for the opportunities or you may find that all your attention is going to the baby without you even realizing it.

You'll also realize that you begin to feel differently about each other. This doesn't mean less, just different. It isn't a sign that your relationship is deteriorating; it is more likely to mature and become

Make the most of your new baby
Relationships begin in the early days and weeks of your new baby's life. Make sure you have as much time with him as possible to build on it.

richer. Don't keep wishing that it was the same as before, because it never can be.

Adjustment to fatherhood

If you're relaxed and confident about the newborn baby, you'll enjoy family life much more and your involvement will help you to appreciate that looking after a baby is every bit as exhausting as a day at work.

• Start bathing and changing your baby as soon as possible.

• Spend as much time as you can with your baby and make sure you have him to yourself on a regular basis – your partner will be glad of the break.

• Talk to your employers about your new baby. If you have to get away early or adopt more flexible working hours for a while, they may be more amenable if they've been warned and you will know where you stand in relation to paternity leave (*see p.249*).

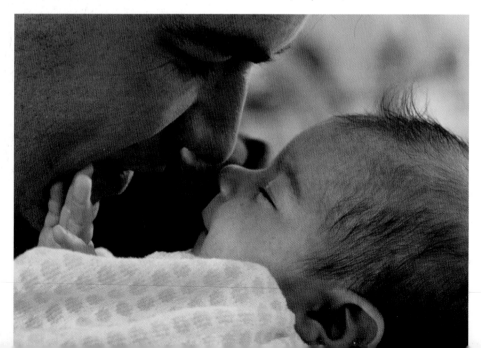

Meeting other children

If you have another child (or children) and are not having your baby at home, it is worth thinking carefully about how you are going to introduce your child to a new baby and so help to avoid jealousy. When you first greet him, make sure that someone else is carrying the baby so that your arms are free to hold out, welcome him and gather him up for a cuddle. For the first few minutes give him all your attention, just as you would if you had been apart for any other reason.

Bring a present from the newborn baby – something that your child has really been looking forward to having. If possible, let him hold the newborn baby himself. Most young children are anxious to be of help, so encourage your child to give you all the assistance he can. During the first days and weeks, set aside some times, several each day if you can, which are just for you and him to be together.

Continue child's special routines

Don't break old habits just because the new baby has come. So, if you always had a special morning or evening routine, continue it with your child if you possibly can. Feed the baby just before these special times, so you won't be interrupted. When you have visitors, don't let them pay all their attention to the newborn baby and ignore your older child. It also helps if you can praise and reward your child as much as you can in the first few weeks. If you're going to be in hospital for several days, try to make arrangements for your child to come into hospital to see you and the baby as soon as possible after delivery and regularly thereafter.

TIPS FOR COPING WITH TIREDNESS

Even if your baby sleeps well between feeds, your body needs to recover from the birth, and you will feel tired, particularly in the afternoon. To keep up your strength and good spirits and to get back to normal quickly, get as much rest as you can.

- Have a rest whenever the baby is sleeping; don't use his sleep time for chores.
- If you aren't feeling well, don't be stoical, call your doctor; your health could get worse.
- Continue to take any prescribed iron pills for at least six weeks after the birth.
- Keep to the balanced diet you had during pregnancy (see pp.106–114) and pay particular attention to what you eat if you are breast-feeding your baby. This is not the time to diet. Breast-feeding in itself uses up fat laid down for the purpose during pregnancy.
- Drink lots of fluids; you will feel very thirsty if you are breast-feeding.
- Have meals and snacks that require the minimum of preparation such as salads, cheese, cold meat sandwiches made with wholemeal bread, fresh fruit and yogurt.
- Take all the short cuts you can think of.
- Accept any offers of help for cooking and cleaning, so that you can relax and enjoy time with the baby and get some rest.
- Let your older children help with the baby – tidying the cot or putting away the nappies.
- Keep the baby in the room with you for the first few weeks. You won't have to go far to pick him up and you can sit up in bed to feed him.
- Keep a couple of nappies in the kitchen, the car and the bathroom as well as the baby's room, so you don't have to go back to the baby's room for every nappy change.
- Believe in the fact that you need help and accept any offers you get.

Making love again

Your relationship with your partner changes in all sorts of ways and for most people this includes sex. Some women lose their sex drive for a couple of months after childbirth and sometimes for longer. Some fathers feel the same and lose their ability to maintain an erection. If you both can be philosophical and loving about your problems, you'll prevent them developing into long-term obstacles.

When to resume sex

There is no magic date when you can start to have sexual relations again. It will help if you start your pelvic floor exercises (*see p.123*) immediately after delivery, even if you're a bit sore. Take it slowly and gently. The ideal time to start making love again is when you and your partner want to, so discuss it and try it out tentatively. You may find that the tissues are a bit sore or tight, but waiting will not make them stretch. Glands that normally lubricate the vaginal area sometimes don't function for a short while after delivery, so use a lubricating cream or jelly. It helps, too, if the vagina is well relaxed before penetration, so concentrate on foreplay. Try a different position from the woman lying on her back as the penis can press on the rear wall of the vagina, which may still be sensitive and slightly bruised. Don't be concerned about set-backs – they're normal; try again gently.

If you've had an episiotomy you'll be sore and tender for longer and your partner should not attempt penetration until you feel comfortable. However, don't let this rule out gentle exploration.

If after several months one of you is still feeling reluctant about sex, do ask for help. You'll be surprised how much easier it is once you've talked to someone, and it may be easier for you both to talk with a third party, perhaps a friend or a sex counsellor. The most important thing is to talk about your feelings.

LOSS OF LIBIDO

- Many women feel unattractive for a while after childbirth; your body will still be a bit shapeless compared to your pre-pregnancy figure. It's difficult to feel sexually attractive if you have a poor self-image (*see p.100*).
- The presence of the baby may be a stumbling block to expressions of love and sexual interest, especially if he is sleeping in the same room.
- You'll both be tired, which does tend to inhibit your libido. Try to rest as much as possible.
- Particularly if you had an episiotomy or a Caesarean, your scar will take a while to heal and you may be loathe to try having sex for the time being.
- Parents do become very baby-orientated in the first few weeks, and you may feel that there isn't room for anyone else in your emotions. This is perfectly natural. What you should do is tell your partner about your feelings. You'll probably both feel this way to some degree.
- Many of the daily activities surrounding babies may make you feel unattractive – washing nappies, and smells of posset – all these things can be a bit off-putting.

CONTRACEPTION

Even if you are breast-feeding, or haven't restarted menstruating, you are unprotected and should use some form of contraception when you resume intercourse. If you breast-feed your baby totally, your periods will probably not return until you wean him; if you don't breast-feed, or breast-feed only for a short time, your periods should return between two and four months.

You will be asked before you are discharged from hospital about your planned form of contraception and you may want to organize it at this time rather than wait until your postnatal check-up, which is usually between four and six weeks after the birth.

The pill

The contraceptive pill is not usually prescribed until three weeks after the birth of your baby. If you are breast-feeding, the combined pill is not suitable as it contains oestrogen, that can interfere with your metabolism and disrupt your flow of milk.

You can, however, take the progesterone-only, or "mini-pill", which contains no oestrogen and only small amounts of progesterone. The mini-pill is not 100 per cent reliable, you must take one pill every day at around the same time to be sure, but combined with the contraceptive effect of full breast-feeding it should be effective. A tiny amount of the hormone contained in the pill does enter your breast-milk, but current opinion is that the quantities are too small to do any harm to your baby. One study suggests that even if you took the mini-pill for two years while breast-feeding daily, your baby would only absorb the equivalent of one tablet.

During your pregnancy and after the birth you may have suffered certain conditions for the first time. You would be unwise to start using the contraceptive pill after the birth if you have a condition such as high blood pressure, diabetes or postnatal depression.

Cap or diaphragm

You will have to be fitted for a new, larger cap as your old one will no longer be reliable. Use it in conjunction with a spermicidal cream or jelly. You will not be fitted for a new cap until your postnatal check-up, about six weeks after the birth. You should have the size checked again at around six to nine months in case you need another change in size. If you're happy with it, this method is ideal for the somewhat sporadic lovemaking of new parents.

Condom (sheath)

This is the easiest method to use before your check-up. Use plenty of spermicidal jelly or cream with the condom as your vagina will be less well lubricated.

Intrauterine contraceptive device (IUCD)

An IUCD can be inserted at your postnatal check-up. The insertion of an IUCD is much easier once you've had a baby. This is what used to be called a coil.

Mirena device

This hormone-releasing device, inserted like an IUCD, gives five years of contraception and reduces periods. It can be put in at your postnatal visit.

Injections

There is a contraceptive injection available that is recommended by the manufacturers for women who are forgetful. Having been involved in research into these injections, I know some women may have problems with breakthrough bleeding and a return to fertility after three months is not guaranteed for everyone.

Implants

These are long-lasting contraceptives that are inserted under the skin of the forearm. Implanon is an example of this type of contraception.

Postnatal check-up

Your check-up is usually done about six weeks after delivery at a postnatal clinic at the hospital or at your doctor's surgery. The purpose of this check-up is to give you a thorough medical and obstetric examination to make sure everything has returned to normal. Your baby is also checked at six weeks, either at a special baby clinic or at your doctor's surgery. If there was any cause for concern at birth you may be asked to bring your baby back to the hospital for his check-up.

When you go for your check-up, take the chance to ask about anything that's bothering you, sort out problems and seek reassurance about things that may be causing you anxiety. These questions may be about your baby, your own well-being, sex, feeding, crying, routines – anything that you feel needs clarifying.

During your own medical check-up your blood pressure will be measured and your weight will be noted, your nipples and breasts will be examined, your abdomen will be palpated to check that the uterus has contracted down to its pre-pregnant size, and you'll have an internal examination and a smear test. If you're suffering from any bladder discomfort or pain when you move your bowels, tell your doctor. Talk again about contraception too (*see p.235*). A perfect time to have an IUCD or a diaphragm fitted is during the internal examination. The doctor will also check your scar if you had any stitching.

The baby's six-week check

It is usual for the baby to be weighed and to have his eyes, cord, genitalia and skin checked and for you to have a general discussion with the health visitor or doctor about how feeding is going. This would be the time to raise any queries you might have about the daily care of the baby and what you might expect to happen over the next few weeks and months.

Going back to work

Even if you committed yourself to going back to work while you were pregnant (*see p.30*), you may now want to rethink your decision, depending on your emotional and financial circumstances. You should also consult your doctor, who can advise you about factors affecting your health and that of the baby. You should start finding a good system of childcare about six weeks before you intend to return to work, and

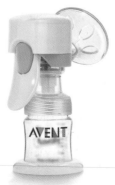

Expressing breast-milk
Modern breast pumps make expressing much easier. Some electric ones have an electronic memory to record your particular pumping rhythm.

begin weaning your baby off the breast then, too, at least during the day.

If you begin working before your baby is four months old, and therefore while you are still breast-feeding, you will need to plan. Try to introduce a routine so that feeding times are predictable and constant. Feed your baby at breakfast and around 6pm; then the person who looks after him need give only the expressed milk or milk substitute for the other two daytime feeds.

If you don't want your baby to take any milk substitutes, freeze expressed breast-milk; it will keep for up to six months in the freezer. It should take around two weeks to get into this routine. You will need to run down your daytime milk production before you return to work or you'll find that your breasts will feel most uncomfortable during the day.

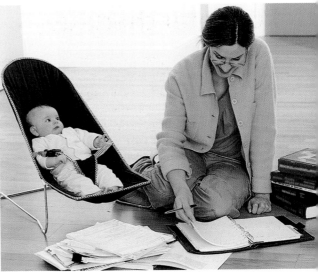

Working from home
If you are lucky enough to have freelance work in your own home, your baby can stay with you. You may need some help with childcare once he is more wakeful.

Finding good childcare

Ask around your friends, neighbours, the local council and independent groups to find out what kind of childcare is available in your area. The options may include:
- Childminders – women who look after children in their own homes. Ask your local authority for a list or take the advice of your health visitor. Always visit a childminder a few times before you put your baby or child into her care.
- Day nurseries – these are run privately or by local authorities. Private day nurseries may be quite expensive; local authority nurseries may have long waiting lists.

Both usually have only a limited number of places for young babies.
- Nannies – usually young women with a nursery nurses' qualification. They may live in or come to your home on a daily basis. Trained nannies are often the most reliable option for mothers returning to work full-time, especially while their babies are still young.
- Mother's helps or au pairs – untrained girls and young women who live with you and help with childcare, babysitting and light housework. They should not be expected to take on the sole care of a young baby for any length of time.
- Workplace crèches – these can be ideal, particularly if you want to continue to breast-feed after you return to work. Unfortunately they are still rare.

Enjoying parenthood

I've spoken to many mothers who feel that they've reached the end of their tether within the first few weeks of having a baby. It's important for you to release your pent-up feelings and ease tension and anxiety and enjoy being a parent.

- You really don't have to worry about giving babycare a high priority, you automatically will. You do have to make an effort, though, to give care of yourself a higher priority than most reasonable women want to do. Try to be a little more selfish than you want to be by replacing the less important babycare activities with care of yourself. Your ultimate aim should be your own peace of mind and happiness. This is particularly important if you are breast-feeding; it is essential that you are fit and rested.
- Even in the early days when you're drawn to be with your baby most of the time, it's essential to have some time on your own, so do whatever you have to

do to get it. Perhaps you could arrange with a friend to leave your baby with her for an afternoon a week, and you can do the same for her. You might like to make this a permanent arrangement.

- Don't isolate yourself for too long. Often during the early weeks, you may feel agoraphobic and want to keep safe inside the house with your baby, away from traffic noise and the outside world. If this is your first child, you will soon build up a circle of contacts, either through an independent group or by making friends with other women in the hospital. You could also join or set up a babysitting circle in your area.
- Find out about the playgroups and community centres in your area and see what they have to offer. There may be crèche facilities while you attend a dance class or discussion group or go shopping.
- Don't expect too much of yourself or of your baby. You aren't perfect, but neither

COPING WITH CRYING

Babies sleep a lot during the first few months, but they also cry a lot as well. Crying is their only means of communication and may be for any number of causes. Check the following:
- Is he hungry? Even if he only fed two hours ago, he might want some more.
- Check his nappy; it could be uncomfortably wet or dirty.
- Is his room warm enough or is he too hot (or too cold)? Babies need a constant temperature of about 18–20°C (65–68°F). If he is too hot, remove some of the covers.

- He may be bored and lonely and want company.
- If your baby mainly cries for prolonged periods at a particular time of day – especially in the evening – it may be what is often known as "colic". No one quite knows what causes this typical pattern of crying. Typically the baby is difficult to console and may draw his legs up to his chest as though he has a tummyache. Ask your health visitor to advise you on the best way to soothe him – don't hesitate to use a dummy if that helps – and hang on to the fact that babies generally grow out of colic by three to four months of age.

is your baby and you have to forgive imperfections in him as well as yourself. Don't set impossibly high standards of mother or baby behaviour. Be prepared to be as flexible as you possibly can.

• Most people find the first early weeks with a baby scary. I did with each of my children and longed for reassurance from the midwife. What you can rely on is the sure knowledge that mothers have taken care of their infants instinctively for millennia, and you are endowed with the same abilities as those mothers.

Meeting other new mothers
Talking to other new parents can open up a new circle of friends. You will also find comfort in talking to other parents about looking after young babies.

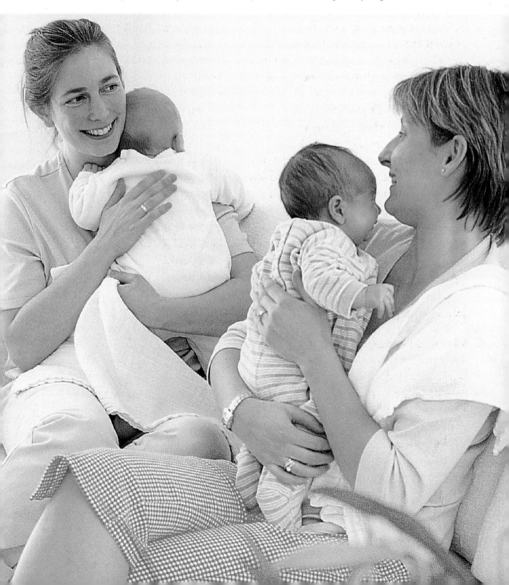

Writing a birthplan

The nine months of your pregnancy will be a time of decision making and preparation for you and your partner. You may already have strong views about how your labour and birth should be managed, or you may want to be guided by friends who have already had babies and the medical staff who are caring for you.

Name: Annette Gale
Doctor: Dr. Carrington
Midwife: Sally Lord

Birth attendant/coach

My partner very much wants to be present but he feels some trepidation and would prefer not to be the only birth attendant, so I would like my friend Jane to be there too as birth coach. She has had three children herself and is a calm person. I would like one of them to be there throughout.

Pain relief

I would like to try to manage without but would not object to trying a TENS machine. I'd like the use of a birthing pool if available. My partner has practised aromatherapy massage and I would like to try this for the first stage. If I don't feel that I am managing and the labour is going on a long time, please advise me on having pethidine, saving an epidural as a last option.

Managing labour

I really want to walk around so please don't link me to a belt monitor unless it is medically necessary for the safety of my baby. I would like to arrange to bring in some big cushions to lean on during labour. My two birth attendants can perhaps support me at times.

Position for birth

I really want to squat to deliver. That is why my friend Jane could be so useful as she and my partner could hold me on either side. I haven't tried a birthing stool but if you had one, I could try that. If I'm too tired, I'd like to deliver on all fours on the floor or on the bed.

Birthplan

There are a number of choices to be made (*see pp.53–67*), and once you have considered the issues and decided what sort of birth you would ideally like, you can write them down in note form on a birthplan, which is kept with your notes. Don't worry if you change your mind, as your birthplan can be amended.

There is no guarantee that everything will go exactly as you expect during your labour and birth, and it's helpful to discuss your approach with the midwife or doctor at the clinic so that they can support you in your decision. During labour you're unlikely to be thinking clearly so make sure your partner understands your birthplan, and reminds staff about it. If you don't know the midwife who attends your labour, check that she has seen your birthplan. Below is a sample birthplan as a guide.

Birthplan

Medical routines
If I have to be induced, I would prefer if it could done by first trying prostaglandin pessaries, then by rupturing the membranes. If these do not speed things up, I'll take medical advice but I would prefer not to be induced by intravenous drip. I didn't tear last time so I'd prefer not to have an episiotomy unless forceps are needed.

The birth
I regretted not putting my hand down last time to touch the baby's head, so I would like to do that this time. Could you let me know when it appears? Then please put my baby on my tummy afterwards. I do not object to the injected drug that speeds up the third stage.

Breastfeeding
I would like to put the baby to my breast as soon as possible. If the baby has to go to a special unit for any reason, I would want to express milk and get breastfeeding going.

Unforeseen problems
- If I have to have an emergency Caesarean, can my husband hold the baby until I'm able to?
- If the labour is long and I am tiring or the baby is becoming distressed, I will be happy for you to accelerate labour.

Notes
- If I have to stay in hospital, I would like my mother and Thomas, my two-year-old, to be able to visit at any time.
- Please note that I am vegetarian.

Useful addresses

Labour and birth

The Active Birth Centre
25 Bickerton Road
London N19 5JT
020 7281 6760
www.activebirthcentre.com
Information and classes if you want to avoid a high-tech birth.

Action on Pre-eclampsia
2c The Halfcroft
Syston LE7 1LD
020 8863 3271
www.apec.org.uk
Advice on pre-eclampsia.

AcuMedic
101–105 Camden High Street
London NW1 7JN
020 7388 6704
www.acumedic.com
Acupuncture and fertility.

Association of Radical Midwives
16 Wytham Street
Oxford OX1 4SU
01865 248 159
www.radmid.demon.co.uk
Supports women and midwives in their choices for childbirth.

British Liver Trust
2 Southampton Road
Ringwood BH24 1HY
0870 652 7330 (Helpline)
www.britishlivertrust.org.uk

Provides Information and advice on liver disease in pregnancy.

Independent Midwives' Association
PO Box 539
Abingdon
Oxon OX14 9DF
0845 4600 105
www.independentmidwives.org.uk
Network of independent midwives offering private care.

National Childbirth Trust
Alexandra House
Oldham Terrace
London W3 6NH
0870 4448707
www.nct.org.uk
Organizes antenatal classes and offers help after a baby is born.

Royal College of Midwives
15 Mansfield Street
London W1G 9NH
020 7312 3535
www.rcm.org.uk

Royal College of Obstetricians & Gynaecologists
27 Sussex Place
London NW1 4RG
020 7772 6200
www.rcog.org.uk
Provides lists of obstetricians.

Breastfeeding

Association of Breastfeeding Mothers
PO Box 207
Bridgwater
TA6 7YT
0870 401 7711
08444 122 929 (counselling hotline)
www.abm.me.uk

La Leche League (Great Britain)
PO Box 29
West Bridgford
Nottingham NG2 7NP
0845 120 2918 (helpline)
www.laleche.org.uk
Help and information for mothers who want to breastfeed.

Parent Support

The Association for Postnatal Illness
145 Dawes Road
London SW6 7EB
020 7386 0868
www.apni.org

BLISS (Baby Life Support Systems)
2nd & 3rd Floors
9 Holyrood Street
London SE1 2EL
0500 618 140 (helpline)
www.bliss.org.uk
Helpline for parents of special-care babies.

The Compassionate Friends
53 North Street
Bristol BS3 1EN
0845 123 2304 (helpline)
www.tcf.org.uk
Puts bereaved parents in touch with others.

Contact a Family
209–211 City Road
London EC1V 1JN
020 7608 8700
0808 808 3555 (helpline)
www.cafamily.org.uk
Puts parents of children with special needs in touch with others.

CRY-SIS Support Group
BM Cry-Sis
London WC1N 3XX
08451 228 669
Advice for parents about crying babies.

The Foundation for the Study of Infant Deaths
11–19 Artillery Row
London SW1P 1RT
020 7222 8001
020 7233 2090 (helpline)
www.sids.org.uk
Researches the causes of SIDS and provides support.

Gingerbread: One parent families
255 Kentish Town Road
London NW5 2LX
0800 018 5026 (helpline)
www.oneparent

familes.org.uk.
Support for one-parent families.

Home-Start
2 Salisbury Road
Leicester LE1 7QR
0800 068 63 68
www.home-start.org.uk
Information and support in the home for parents with at least one child under five.

Infertility Network UK
Charter House
43 St Leonards Road
Bexhill-on-Sea
East Sussex TN40 1JA
0800 008 7464
www.infertilitynetworkuk.com
Information, support and advice for people who experience infertility.

The Miscarriage Association
c/o Clayton Hospital
Northgate, Wakefield
West Yorkshire WF1 3JS
01924 200799
www.miscarriage
association.org.uk
Support for after a miscarriage.

The National Meet-a-Mum Association (MAMA)
54 Lillington Road
Radstock BA3 3NR
0845 120 3746
www.mama.co.uk

Help for new mothers, particularly with postnatal depression.

Parentline Plus
520 Highgate Studios
53–79 Highgate Road
London NW5 1TL
0808 800 2222 (helpline)
www.parentlineplus.org.uk
Support for parents and carers.

Stillbirth and Neonatal Death Society (SANDS)
28 Portland Place
London W1B 1LY
020 7436 5881 (helpline)
www.uk-sands.org

St Mary's Hospital Recurrent Miscarriage Clinic
Winston Churchill Wing
Praed Street
London W2 1NY
020 7886 6000
www.st-marys.nhs.uk

Twins and Multiple Births Association (TAMBA)
2 The Willows
Gardner Road
Guildford
Surrey
GU1 4PG
0800 138 0509 (twinline)
www.tamba.org.uk
A self-help organization offering encouragement and support before and after multiple births.

Children with special needs

Association for Spina Bifida and Hydrocephalus (ASBAH)
Asbah House
42 Park Road
Peterborough PE1 2UQ
0845 450 7755
www.asbah.org
Information and advice for parents of children with spina bifida.

Down's Syndrome Association
Langdon Down Centre
2a Langdon Park
Teddington TW11 9PS
0845 230 0372
www.downs-syndrome.org.uk
Advice on the care and treatment of children with Down's syndrome.

MENCAP
123 Golden Lane
London EC1Y 0RT
020 7454 0454
www.mencap.org.uk
Support for families of children with learning difficulties.

Scope
PO Box 833
Milton Keynes
MK12 5NY
(include stamped addressed envelope if you write)
0800 800 3333
www.scope.org.uk

Information and support for children with cerebral palsy and their families.

Sickle Cell Society
54 Station Road
London NW10 4UA
020 8961 7795
www.sicklecellsociety.org
Information about sickle cell disease.

Family planning

British Pregnancy Advisory Service (BPAS)
20 Timothy's Bridge Road
Stratford Enterprise Park
Stratford-Upon-Avon
Warwick CV37 9BF
08457 304030 (information line)
www.bpas.org
Advice on contraception.

Brook
421 Highgate Studios
51–79 Highgate Road
London NW5 1TL
020 7950 7700 (24-hour information line)
www.brook.org.uk
Advice on contraception and pregnancy testing.

fpa (The Family Planning Association)
50 Featherstone Street
London EC1Y 8QU
0845 122 8690 (helpline)
www.fpa.org.uk

Marie Stopes House Family Planning Clinic
108 Whitfield Street
London WIT 5BE
0845 300 8090 (24-hour helpline)
www.mariestopes.org.uk
Information and advice about family planning, sterilization etc.

Complementary medicine

British Acupuncture Council
63 Jeddo Road
London W12 9HQ
020 8735 0400
www.acupuncture.org.uk
Provides a list of practitioners.

British Homeopathic Association
Hahnemann House
29 Park Street West
Luton LU1 3BE
0870 444 3950
www.trusthomeopathy.org

British Medical Acupuncture Society (BMAS)
BMAS House
3 Winnington Court
Winnington Street
Northwich
Cheshire CW8 1AQ
01606 786782
www.medical-acupuncture.co.uk
Provides membership lists.

**Institute for
Complementary Medicine**
Can-Mezzanine
32–36 Loman Street
London SE1 0EH
www.i-c-m.org.uk
*Provides information on
complementary medicine.*

General
**Association for
Improvements
in Maternity Services
(AIMS)**
5 Ann's Court
Grove Road
Surbiton KT6 4BE
0870 765 1433 (helpline)
www.aims.org.uk
*Provides support and information
about maternity choices.*

**Child Accident
Prevention Trust**
4th Floor
Cloister Court
22–26 Farringdon Lane
London EC1R 3AJ
020 7608 3828
www.capt.org.uk
*Advice on avoiding childhood
accidents and injuries.*

The Lady
39–40 Bedford Street
London WC2E 9ER
020 7379 4717
www.lady.co.uk
*Magazine with advertisements
for childcarers.*

**National Childminding
Association**
Royal Court
81 Tweedy Road
Bromley
Kent BR1 1TG
0845 880 0044
www.ncma.org.uk
*Organization of those interested
in pre-school care of babies and
children and to improve the
status of minders and the
facilities for the children.*

**Recruitment and
Employment
Services**
15 Welbeck Street
London
W1G 9XT
020 7009 2100
www.rec.co.uk
*Send SAE for a list of
nanny agencies.*

Vegan Society
Donald Watson House
21 Hylton Street
Hockley, Birmingham
B18 6HJ
0121 523 1730
www.vegansociety.com
Information and advice on diets.

Wellbeing
27 Sussex Place
London NW1 4SP
020 7772 6400
www.wellbeingofwomen.
org.uk
Funds research for better health

*for women and babies and
development of new treatments
for problems during and after
the birth.*

Women's Health Concern
4–6 Eton Place
Marlow
Buckinghamshire SL7 2QA
0845 123 2319 (helpline)
www.womens-health-
concern.org
*Offers advice on all
gynaecological problems and
health queries.*

Further reading

Miriam Stoppard
Baby First Aid
Dorling Kindersley 2003

Baby's First Skills
Dorling Kindersley 2009

Conception, Pregnancy and Birth
Dorling Kindersley 2008

Complete Baby & Childcare
Dorling Kindersley 2008

First-Time Parents
Dorling Kindersley 2009

New Babycare
Dorling Kindersley 2009

Bonding with your Bump
Dorling Kindersley 2008

My Pregnancy Planner
Dorling Kindersley 2007

DK Healthcare: You and Your Toddler
Dorling Kindersley 2006

Yehudi Gordon
Birth and Beyond
Vermilion 2002

Erika Lenkert
The Real Deal Guide to Pregnancy
Dorling Kindersley 2008

Catharine Parker-Littler
Ask a Midwife
Dorling Kindersley 2008

The British Red Cross
First Aid for Babies and Children Fast
Dorling Kindersley 2006

Dr Jane Collins, Great Ormond Street Hospital
Children's Medical Guide
Dorling Kindersley 2007

Dr Carol Cooper
Johnson's Mother and Baby
Dorling Kindersley 2006

Twins and Multiple Births
Vermilion 1997

Baby and Child Questions and Answers
Dorling Kindersley 2006

Arlene Eisenberg
What to Expect When You're Expecting
Simon and Schuster 2002

Elizabeth Fenwick
Healthy Pregnancy (101 Essential Tips)
Dorling Kindersley 2004

Dr Richard Ferber
Solve Your Child's Sleep Problems
Dorling Kindersley 2006

Francoise Barbira Freedman
Yoga for Pregnancy, Birth & Beyond
Dorling Kindersley 2004

Dr Alan Heath and Nicki Bainbridge
Baby Massage
Dorling Kindersley 2004

Sheila Kitzinger
New Pregnancy and Childbirth
Dorling Kindersley 2008

Birth Your Way
Dorling Kindersley 2002

Birth Crisis
Routledge 2006

Dr Christoph Lees, Grainne McCartan
Pregnancy Questions & Answers
Dorling Kindersley 2007

Penelope Leach
Your Baby & Child
Dorling Kindersley 2003

Hope Ricciotti
*The Yummy Mummy
Pregnancy Cookbook*
Dorling Kindersley 2007

Margot Sunderland
The Science of Parenting
Dorling Kindersley 2006

Zita West
Plan to Get Pregnant
Dorling Kindersley 2008

Babycare before Birth
Dorling Kindersley 2006

Lesley Regan
*Your Pregnancy Week-by-
Week*
Dorling Kindersley 2005

Your rights and benefits

Pregnant women are entitled to a range of rights and benefits depending on their circumstances and National Insurance (NI) contributions. The entitlements, particularly for those on low incomes, are complicated, but your Social Security office, Citizen's Advice Bureau or legal advice centre should be able to advise you and work out what you are eligible for.

If you are in paid employment, any maternity leave and pay from your employer must be explained to you by your employer or trade union representative. The chart overleaf shows you how to get your maximum entitlement. If you need further information, contact your local Social Security office or Job Centre.

Benefits during pregnancy

Pregnant women are eligible for free NHS dental treatment and prescriptions, and you may get free milk and vitamins if you are on a low income. Statutory Maternity Pay (SMP) is operated by your employer and is not dependent on your going back to work. For pregnant women who can't get SMP because they are self-employed, have changed jobs or are not working, there is a Maternity Allowance payable for up to 26 weeks provided the qualifying conditions are satisfied.

If you are not entitled to SMP or Maternity Allowance, you may get eight weeks' incapacity benefit. Mothers who are on Income Support or Family Credit, may get a maternity payment from the Social Fund. Women on their own after the baby is born get a tax-free weekly cash payment (on top of child benefit) regardless of income or NI contributions.

Working women

As an employee, you are entitled by law to 52 weeks' maternity leave, however long you have worked for your employer. During this time you are entitled to all your normal terms of employment except wages or salary, and afterwards you can return to your job. The earliest you can start your leave is 11 weeks before the week that you expect your baby.

To qualify for SMP you must have been in the same employment for at least 26 weeks without a break by the 15th week before the week your baby is due, and you must have earned enough to pay Class 1 NI contributions. SMP is paid for up to 26 weeks. For the first six weeks you get 90 per cent of your average weekly earnings and a flat rate after that. SMP may be liable to the normal deductions from your wages.

On top of that, Additional Maternity Leave lasts for 26 weeks and starts at the end of Ordinary Maternity Leave. You are entitled to Additional Maternity Leave if you have worked for your employer for 26 weeks by the 14th week before your baby is due. It is important that you tell your employer what you are going to do, and make it clear if you wish to return to work so your job is kept open for you. You are also entitled to paid time off to go to your

WHEN	WHAT TO DO	WHY
As soon as you know you are pregnant	1 Ask your doctor for form FW8. 2 Tell your dentist. 3 Check leaflet HC 11 and tell your Social Security office if you are getting Income Support. 4 Tell your employer. 5 Find out about Maternity Allowance.	1 To apply for free prescriptions. 2 To get free dental treatment. 3 To check your right to free glasses, free milk and vitamins, and help with hospital fares. 4 To find out about Statutory Maternity Pay (SMP) and time off for antenatal appointments. 5 If you can't get SMP.
As soon as you can	If you are unemployed or ill, ask your Social Security office about making a claim for Maternity Allowance.	It can affect the amount of Maternity Allowance you may get.
20 weeks of pregnancy	1 Ask your doctor or midwife for a maternity certificate (form MAT B1) showing when your baby is due. 2 If you are employed, give the MAT B1 form to your employer. 3 If you cannot get SMP, ask at your maternity or child health clinic or Social Security office for form MA 1.	1 You need this form to qualify for SMP or Maternity Allowance. 2 To protect your right to SMP and allow your employer to work out your entitlement. If you delay later than three weeks after your SMP could have started, you may lose your SMP. 3 You can apply for Maternity Allowance on form MA 1.
At least three weeks before you intend to stop work	Tell your employer in writing when you will be stopping work; the week the baby is due; and whether you intend to return to your job.	To protect your right to SMP, maternity leave and the right to return to work at the end of the longer maternity absence.
29 weeks Your 14 week maternity leave period can start now.	Apply for a maternity payment from the Social Fund if you or your partner are on Income Support, Family Credit or Disability Working Allowance.	To pay for items for the baby.

antenatal clinics and you are protected against unfair dismissal when pregnant.

Paternity leave

A man is eligible for paid paternity leave of one or two weeks after a baby is born provided that he is the biological father of the baby or the mother's partner with responsibility for bringing up the child. He must have been working for his employer for 26 weeks by the 15th week before the baby is due. He must also give his employer at least 28 days' notice of when he would like paternity leave to start.

WHEN	WHAT TO DO	WHY
As soon after the birth as possible	1 Register the baby's birth. This must be done within 6 weeks (3 weeks in Scotland). 2 Send off form for Child Benefit and, if you are a single parent, for Lone Parent payment. 3 Ask about low income benefits.	1 To get the birth certificate and NHS card. 2 To get Child Benefit and Lone Parent payment. 3 To see if you qualify for extra income support; help with rent, council tax, dental treatment and hospital fares; and free prescriptions, milk and vitamins.
During your maternity leave	1 Give your employer 28 days' notice if you want to go back to work before the end of your 52 weeks' maternity leave. If you want to go back to work at the end of 52 weeks' maternity leave, you do not need to do anything. 2 Reply in writing within two weeks to any letter from your employer asking if you are going back to work after the end of the longer maternity.	1 Your employer can postpone your return for up to seven days if you do not tell them you want to go back early. 2 To protect your right to return to work by the end of the 28th week after the week your baby is born.
3 months after the birth	If you or your partner are getting Income Support or Family Credit, apply for a maternity payment from the Social Fund.	You will lose maternity payment from the Social Fund if not claimed by now.
3 weeks before return to work	Write to your employer stating that you wish to return.	To protect your right to return to work.
29 weeks from the birth	Return to work as your maternity leave is officially over.	You may lose your right to return to work.
6 months after the birth	Claim Child Benefit.	Latest date for claiming, if Child Benefit is to be paid from date of birth.

Index

Acknowledgments

Medical consultant:
Dr Elizabeth Owen MD FRCOG MHPEd

Cooling Brown would like to thank:
Hilary Bird for the index; Constance Novis for
proofreading; Romaine Werblow for finding the
images in the DK library

Illustrations for new edition Debbie Maizels

The publisher would like to thank the following
for their kind permission to reproduce their
photographs:
(Key: a-above; b-below/bottom; c-centre; l-left;
r-right; t-top)
Photograph of breast pump on page 236
courtesy of Avent Ltd
Alamy Images: David Young-Wolff 218;
Corbis: Cameron 213; Brownie Harris 209, Larry
Williams 9; **Getty Images:** George Doyle 13;
Tom Grill 57; Stockbyte Platinum 13; Phillip &
Karen Smith 218; Nancy Durrell McKenna 57;

Mother & Baby Picture Library: 39, 42br, 44,
50, 105, 139, 155, 171, 174, 190, 216, 225;
Moose Azim 194; Emap elan 35, 37, 39, 41, 43,
45, 47, 49, 51; EMAP Ian Hooton 36, 44, 69,
72, 73bl, 73br, 76c; Ruth Jenkinson 192, 200;
Caroline Molloy 38; Anthea Sieveking 187;
Photolibrary: BananaStock 184; **Science Photo
Library:** AJ Photo 34; BSIP/Astier 78; Tracey
Dominey 205; GE Medical Systems 86, 89; Dr
Najeeb Layyous 85bl; Joseph Nettis 209; ZEPHYR
91; **SuperStock:** 6; **The Wellcome Institute
Library, London:** Anthea Sieveking 1, 2, 55,
171, 183t, 187, 188.

Jacket images: *Front and spine:* Science Photo
Library: Ian Hooton. *Back:* Author Portrait:
Carolyn Djanogly for DK; Alamy Images:
photocay.

All other images © Dorling Kindersley
For further information see:
www.dkimages.com